NEUROSIS IN THE
ORDINARY FAMILY

TAVISTOCK

FAMILIES & MARRIAGE
In 6 Volumes

NEUROSIS IN THE ORDINARY FAMILY

A Psychiatric Survey

ANTHONY RYLE

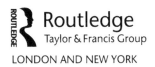

Routledge
Taylor & Francis Group

LONDON AND NEW YORK

First published in 1967 by
Tavistock Publications Limited

Published in 2001 by
Routledge
2 Park Square, Milton Park, Abingdon, Oxfordshire OX14 4RN
711 Third Avenue, New York, NY 10017

First issued in paperback 2014

Routledge is an imprint of the Taylor and Francis Group, an informa business

British Library Cataloguing in Publication Data
A CIP catalogue record for this book
is available from the British Library

Neurosis in the Ordinary Family
ISBN 0-415-26421-9
Families & Marriage: 6 Volumes
ISBN 0-415-26508-8
The International Behavioural and Social Sciences Library
112 Volumes
ISBN 0-415-25670-4

ISBN 13: 978-1-138-88265-2 (pbk)
ISBN 13: 978-0-415-26421-1 (hbk)

Neurosis in the Ordinary Family

A PSYCHIATRIC SURVEY

ANTHONY RYLE, D.M.

Foreword by D. A. Pond, M.D., F.R.C.P., D.P.M.
Professor of Psychiatry,
The London Hospital Medical College

TAVISTOCK PUBLICATIONS

J. B. LIPPINCOTT COMPANY

First published in Great Britain in 1967
by Tavistock Publications Ltd
2 Park Square, Milton Park, Abingdon,
Oxon, OX14 4RN
in 11 point Times New Roman
by Ebenezer Baylis & Son, The Trinity Press
Worcester and London

Distributed in the United States of America
and in Canada by J. B. Lippincott Company
Philadelphia and Toronto

In memory of
Angus McPherson, neurophysiologist
who helped me to go on thinking

Contents

Foreword

This book is a contribution to the rapidly growing literature of epidemiological studies in mental disorder. It has taken some time for psychiatrists trained in medicine to get away from hospital-based studies and crude concepts of mental disease as clinical entities to a more biological approach to the study of human disorder in its natural habitat, which is emphatically not a hospital ward or an outpatient department. This work must be seen in the first place as an essay in methodology, for there is a rich field of study into what is worth looking at and what is not. That there were not many more mistakes made is entirely due to the author's skill in choosing the best possible investigatory tools, and to the skill of Miss Madge Hamilton who did the interviewing.

The study of family patterns of behaviour provides the essential background for assessing the disturbances that may present at the clinical level to general practitioners, to hospitals or in other ways, such as at school or in delinquency. The interests of psychiatrists are pushing steadily further back in the development of personalities. It might perhaps have been better, as regards the origins of mental disorders, to concentrate on the family of the pre-school child rather than on that of the school child, but it is easy to be wise after the event. This work has been one of the most exciting and instructive investigations I have ever had the pleasure of being associated with, and I hope that others will find it equally stimulating and informative.

D. A. Pond

Acknowledgements

This book was written by a single author, who is responsible for its presentation, but it should be emphasized not only that the work was carried out by a team of three (Dr Pond, Miss Hamilton, and myself) but also that the development of the author's views owes a great deal to the experience of working and exchanging ideas with his more experienced colleagues.

Many people were consulted in the early stages of the project, although it may seem in retrospect that more should have been. Among those who gave us much useful advice I should like in particular to acknowledge the help given by Dr A. N. Oppenheim (London School of Economics) and by Mrs Pat Patten. To Dr Ian Sutherland and Miss Ruth Tall (Medical Research Council Statistical Research Unit) we owe thanks for guiding our statistically naïve minds through our results towards some significant findings, and for the hours of work put into the many calculations that were beyond our skills. We are also grateful to the London County Council Education Department (now the Inner London Education Authority) for permission to approach the schools, and to the very numerous busy teachers who found time to complete forms on the children. We are, of course, very grateful to the 112 families for their co-operation in the survey, and for allowing us to intrude into their lives. The Mental Health Research Fund made the project possible by providing for Miss Hamilton's salary and two sessions weekly for myself, and for the other research expenditure. Finally, I should like to thank Mrs Pat Corbett and Miss Ann Smith for their secretarial assistance at various stages of the project, and to acknowledge the debt owed to Miss Shirley Lesser for her very efficient organization

Acknowledgements

and secretarial assistance throughout. Thanks are due to the publishers and others concerned for permission to quote from the works listed below:

Constable and Company in respect of the excerpt from *An introduction to the study of experimental medicine* by Claude Bernard, translated by H. C. Green; Mr Alexander Dru in respect of passages from his translation of *The journals of Kierkegaard* published by Oxford University Press; Harvard University Press in respect of passages from *The works of Hippocrates*, translated by W. H. S. Jones (Loeb Classical Library edition); The Editor of the *Journal of Child Psychology and Psychiatry* in respect of material from the paper by Dr Ryle and his colleagues, 'The prevalence and patterns of psychological disturbance in children of primary age'.

Introduction

. . . phenomena merely express the relations of bodies,
whence it follows that, by dissociating the parts of a whole,
we must make phenomena cease if only because we destroy
the relations. It follows also in physiology that analysis,
which teaches us the properties of isolated elementary parts,
can never give us more than a most incomplete ideal synthesis; just as knowing a solitary man would not bring us
knowledge of all the institutions which result from man's
association, and which can reveal themselves only through
social life. In a word, when we unite physiological elements,
properties appear which were imperceptible in the separate
elements. We must, therefore, always proceed experimentally
in vital synthesis, because quite different phenomena may
result from more and more complex union or association of
organized elements. All this proves that these elements,
though distinct and self-dependent, do not therefore play the
part of simple associates. A union expresses more than
addition of their separate properties. I am persuaded that the
obstacles surrounding the experimental study of psychological phenomena are largely due to difficulties of this kind . . .

Claude Bernard, *An introduction to
the study of experimental medicine* (1957)

This book is a report of a study of a group of families carried out by
a psychiatrist (D. A. Pond, M.D., F.R.C.P., D.P.M.), a psychiatric social
worker (Madge Hamilton, A.A.P.S.W.), and a general practitioner
(Anthony Ryle, D.M.). The study originated in a suggestion made to
me in 1959 by Dr Pond that a psychiatric social worker might be
placed in my practice to investigate how effectively casework could
be carried out in the setting of a general practice. The difficulties of
designing a satisfactory therapeutic trial, the ethical problem of short-
term treatment intervention, and my own interest in epidemiology, all
led to a modification of this suggestion: the plan finally adopted was
to carry out a survey of a group of families on my National Health

13

Service list, in order to assess the prevalence of emotional disorder. From the point of view of preventive psychiatry, families having children were clearly of particular interest: therefore, to restrict the population size and the number of variables to be allowed for, the study was confined to families with children of primary school age, with a detailed study of the parents, and of the children in that age range. Mental Health Research Fund backing was obtained for the project and we were fortunate in finding, for our team, Madge Hamilton, a psychiatric social worker with previous experience of residential child care, of child guidance, and of family casework with the Canford families (Halmos, 1962). Her family-orientated experience, and her tact, warmth, and skill as an interviewer, added a very valuable dimension to the study.

The first object of the study was to assess the prevalence rates of neurosis and emotional disturbance, a task that had to be done before one could define the scope of work for a psychiatric social worker, or for other therapeutic agencies. In recent years there has been increasing evidence that psychiatric disturbance is far more common in the population than hospital figures and specialist experience suggest. Much of the research which has established this has been based upon general practice which, especially since the start of the National Health Service, has offered unique access to representative groups of the community. The planning of medical education, of general practice, of psychiatry, and particularly of community services, demands a clearer picture of the size and nature of the problem of psychiatric illness than is now available. Our first aim, therefore, was to record the rates of disturbance, using as far as possible more than one means of assessment, and including reproducible objective methods which permitted comparison between our relatively small population and other population groups. In addition to recording the rate of disturbance, we investigated the experience of psychiatrically disturbed individuals in terms of the professional help they had sought and received, recognizing that, particularly in respect of consultation in general practice, there are large variations in the response of doctors.

A second aspect of the work was the investigation of family patterns in neurosis, to discover how far neurosis in one member of the family was associated with its presence in other members, and how far the relationships between family members could be seen to play a

14

part in the production or relief of neurotic symptoms. The central responsibility of the family for transmitting to the child the assumptions and expectations upon which life in society is based, and the family's critical part in determining the individual's chance of attaining maturity and mental health as an adult are unquestioned. How this family influence is exerted, and which variations in the functioning of the family are significantly responsible for different adaptations to different social systems, remain uncertain and in need of investigation.

As well as having a bearing upon aetiological theories, the study of the interaction within the family enabled us to draw some tentative conclusions on the type of professional response which might be provided to lessen the rates of emotional disorder in the community.

The study was medical in orientation, paying particular attention to 'illness' as it is related to the family. However, the concept of illness in psychiatry is to some extent a convenience or a convention (e.g. something that is dealt with by a doctor) rather than a statement of pathology. For example, emotional conflict may be experienced as a conflict, or as a headache, or as a depression, and it may be presented to the doctor, to some other person, or to nobody: and the doctor, if presented with evidence of conflict, may respond to the symptom organically, or psychiatrically, or not at all. These considerations (which are further discussed in Chapter 12) are of considerable practical importance in epidemiology, although Kessel (1960) has shown that comparable estimates of the prevalence of neurotic illness can be derived from the work of practitioners having different orientations, by using a broad, simple definition of disturbance which he labels 'conspicuous psychiatric morbidity'. The criteria of illness used in our study are presented in detail later in the book.

In that part of the study which sought to establish relationships between the family environment and the symptoms of children, we did not rely upon case histories or clinical interpretations. This is not to deny the value of clinical insight, nor to pretend that the observations made were devoid of some theoretical preconceptions. From the point of view of research, however, the most elegant analysis of cases or families in terms of one theory or another cannot provide proof of the correctness of the theory. In treating patients one is of course guided by certain theoretical assumptions. However, the fact that one's assumptions seem to explain the course of events, and

15

possibly even to help the patient, is not evidence of their truth, for practitioners with widely different approaches all manage to find this type of confirmation for their beliefs. The primary method of this study was epidemiological, seeking to demonstrate that certain features and events tend to occur in association in the population. In adopting this method, one has to recognize that the demonstration of an association between two factors is never in itself proof of the presence or the direction of causality. The most definite conclusion that can be drawn from the demonstration of an association is that it is or is not consistent with a particular theory of causation, but even so, this partial form of proof is to be preferred to simple assertion.

In relying upon the demonstration of associations, one is implying that the phenomena studied can be measured. All forms of measurement in psychiatry are inevitably crude, and do scant justice to the complexity of the phenomena. The measures described in the following chapters are of various types and differing reliabilities, in every case falling short of any ideal standard. Details of the methods adopted are provided, and some attempt is made to estimate their validity and reliability. However imperfect they are as tools, they were chosen to eliminate as far as possible any major preconceptions, so it is to be hoped that any associations that have been demonstrated are a function of the phenomena studied, not of the methods of observation.

Good experimental design demands a restriction in the number of variables investigated in any given experiment. However, in dealing with a system with many interdependent variables, all potentially significant, one cannot, in testing the effect of one variable, control for the others without also measuring them. The isolation of a single variable – the ideal technique in research – can often be misleading in psychiatry. For example, the demonstration of an association between maternal deprivation in infancy and subsequent psychological disturbance was probably the most famous example in psychiatry of an epidemiological confirmation of a clinical hypothesis (Bowlby, 1952). Unjustifiable conclusions were often drawn from this work, however, since maternal deprivation has important associated variables which subsequent research has shown to be of at least as much importance as the actual loss of the mother (Ainsworth, 1962; Wootton, 1962; Pringle and Bossio, 1960; Clarke and Clarke, 1960).

Our assessment of the child's environment included a large number of measures, although still all too few in relation to the complexity of the system being studied. We concentrated upon the current state and current relationships of the families, and of necessity ignored both genetic and congenital factors, without denying their importance. Although Miss Hamilton did record a routine developmental history of each child, no attempt was made to relate infant-feeding or toilet-training practices to the child's current adjustment, because there is evidence that parental recollection of these factors is highly unreliable. Other workers have failed to demonstrate significant associations between parents' methods in these areas and the child's later personality (e.g. Sewell, 1952). The data we recorded referred to a number of aspects of the children's current family environment which were considered to be significant in determining psychological health; this information on background, and the descriptions of the children themselves, were made in forms which permitted quantification of the factors.

The information presented in this book refers to individuals, to relationships between pairs, and to family groups. All the families studied contained children and at least one parent. The identification of each family member is given throughout in terms of the relationship of the individual to the child, i.e. as sibling, parent, grandparent, etc. In theory, each individual and the relationship of each individual to every other individual, and to the group as a whole, would be of interest, but our investigation fell far short of this level and dealt in detail with only two sets of relationships: that between mothers and fathers in the marriage relationship, and that between parents and children.

This book contains less material on case histories than the reader might desire. Accounts of casework interviews, and the pictures they paint of people's lives and feelings, are undoubtedly fascinating, but their inclusion would not materially alter the findings or the arguments of the book. Moreover, in so far as interview records clothe the tables and figures with flesh and blood, they also threaten the anonymity of the subjects.[1] Such fragments as are provided are, I believe, sufficiently out of context or, where necessary, sufficiently modified, to prevent their recognition even by the subjects themselves. The ethical problems of publishing case material from anthropological fieldwork has been the subject of a valuable recent article by Barnes

(1963), who argues that a much stricter code is desirable than now applies. In our case there was both a research commitment and a clinical commitment to the families, which imposed an even stronger obligation to respect their confidence. Readers must accept that the families in our study showed the same variety as is found in any group, with anxiety, insecurity, resentment, and need on the one hand, and patience, courage, and resilience on the other.

---

[1] Concern about concealing the identity of individuals has led to the exclusion of a great deal of the case material. Any research worker who wishes to have access to the original survey records is welcome to apply to me.

CHAPTER 1

Methods of Collecting and Recording Data

> For affirmation and talk are deceptive and treacherous,
> wherefore one must . . . occupy oneself with facts persistently
> if one is to acquire that ready and infallible habit which we
> call 'the art of medicine'.
>
> Hippocrates, *Precepts*

> What are called observations are often but a mixture of im-
> perfect observation and unwarranted assumption.
>
> Sir James Mackenzie

Research in social psychiatry depends upon approaching the members of a population for information much of which is private and possibly painful to reveal. Consequently there are both practical and ethical difficulties to be faced in selecting populations for study. Where psychiatric patients or ex-patients are concerned, therapeutic contact has already both provided a measure of information and established rapport. In normal population studies, however, such contact does not exist, and a stranger knocking upon the door cannot reasonably expect or demand detailed information about personality or relationships. One big initial advantage of our study was undoubtedly the fact that, since it was based on my general practice and with my participation, we had both relevant information and rapport established to a considerable degree before the survey, and yet we had a population which was not selected psychiatrically. This privileged access to the population also imposed an obligation not to abuse the confidence established in the general practitioner by in any way forcing the families to co-operate in the research.

I first approached all the families included in the survey through a letter addressed to both parents, explaining that I was taking part in research into children's health and development in relation to the family, offering to call with Miss Hamilton, the social worker, to introduce her and to give further details. A stamped postcard for their reply was enclosed, and a small number of refusals was received at this stage. Where acceptance was expressed, a visit was arranged to explain in more detail the nature of the research, to answer questions about it, and to obtain permission to approach the school for a report upon the children. At this interview care was taken to emphasize the right of the parents to decline to take part. Two or three further refusals were encountered at this stage. The families declining to take part, and a further two or three in which effective co-operation was not achieved owing to repeated postponements or failure to be in at appointed times, contained an above-average number of unhappy marriages, and two cases of recent imprisonment; to this extent, the sample used is less disturbed than the general population registered on my list. In the case of co-operating families, an appointment was made for Miss Hamilton to return for interviewing. Wherever possible this was arranged for a time when both parents could be seen, except for a small number of families in which the father preferred to be left out. In arranging this time, care was taken not to interfere with regular nights out or favoured television programmes.

Three other processes occurred at the time of this interview. Although we had explained in the initial letter that no direct examination of the children was envisaged, in the majority of cases the children were in fact at home and were presented to Miss Hamilton for inspection, a procedure which often threw light on the parents' attitudes. Although this was something we did not systematically record, it was welcome in that it allowed us to explain to the children as well what the survey was about. A second process which often occurred was the use of the visit to address a direct medical request or inquiry to me, a feature possibly representing the need for reassurance that I still fulfilled the role of doctor. The third process was the inspection of Miss Hamilton, a procedure often edged with hostility, apparently aimed at seeing whether she fell into the stereotype of a 'welfare worker' or not. Her ability to weather this inspection, even in the face of parents with long histories of hostility to all patterns of state or voluntary social worker, is a considerable tribute to her skill and personality.

Because of our wish to interview both parents where possible, the majority of interviews were in the evening: however, the mothers were interviewed alone for part of the time in many cases. There are some disadvantages in joint interviewing but, an interview in the home having been decided on, the pattern would have been imposed upon us in most instances by the father's wish to participate. In any case, we soon came to feel that the gain in accuracy and depth from seeing both parents discussing, contradicting, amplifying, and generally interacting, far outweighed any loss. The time spent with each couple averaged about four hours, usually over two interviews, but it varied considerably; the latest interview was continued until well after one o'clock in the morning, but this was fortunately exceptional.

Although the data sheets were planned in detail to cover standard areas on all the families, the interviews themselves were loosely structured, no set order being imposed, and the parents being left to talk spontaneously, or with minimal guidance and prompting wherever possible. Certain areas required more direct questioning than others: for example, the behaviour and symptom profiles of the children could not usually be completed without direct questioning. Interviews were recorded in rough on duplicated sheets, the headings of which provided a check list. At the outset Miss Hamilton would explain that she would have to take notes, and this was accepted and did not seem to create anxiety.

The great majority of parents were frank and forthright in their replies to questions, and ready to give all the necessary information. Conscious distortions or reticence, or the inability fully to comprehend the questions or communicate the replies, were considered to have occurred in only eight families. Most parents became engaged in the research interviews in a way indistinguishable from the casework client in consultation, pouring out doubts, anxieties, and guilt without reserve and often with relief. We had been careful to underline that Miss Hamilton would not return after the research interviews were completed, and that we were concerned to find things out and not to help; and we had stressed that we would not be able to offer continuous support except that already available by my accessibility as the family doctor. Nonetheless, requests for further visits were made by a number of the parents. The fact that parents could be encouraged to consult me in cases of need made Miss Hamilton less anxious about the possible effects of research interviewing than might otherwise have been the case.

Another feature of the interviews was the frequency with which the couple would engage in arguments or discussions about old or previously unexpressed disagreements and disputes. Perhaps the recollections or feelings of one parent, as conveyed at the interview, would provoke the other to present a different version or a different emphasis; or perhaps the presence of a third party would enable one or both to say more directly what had previously been indirectly or only partially expressed. These exchanges were, naturally, often very revealing of the nature of the relationship; they also seemed in many cases to have a beneficial effect and suggested incidentally one of the ways in which a family caseworker might have an impact on the basis of relatively brief intervention. Of all the patients seen by me after their interviews, none had any more hostile observations to make than the few who said, 'I can't see what you want to know all that for.' A larger number were clearly interested and approving of the idea of the research, and many said words to the effect that 'it would be a good thing if everyone had the chance to step back and look at what they're doing every now and then'. A considerable proportion spoke warmly of Miss Hamilton and said it had been a great help to talk to her.

Recording data from an interview with two people lasting four hours or more from relatively brief notes is not easy. Whenever possible it was done soon after the interview, a tape recorder being used to dictate the material in the form required for typing on to record sheets, with duplicated headings, rating scales, and so on. These forms were finalized after the first five interviews, and they included sheets on which information and ratings from my own routine medical notes were recorded, and on which some of the data from questionnaires could also be written. Until these sheets were assembled Miss Hamilton was working 'blind', with no prior knowledge of the families she was interviewing, except in respect of essential information which I let her have before the preliminary visit, such as cases of illegitimacy. Similarly, I recorded data from the general practice records before seeing her notes or discussing the family with her. The arrangement of these sheets is summarized below. The actual rating scales and classifications used, however, are provided in the text where the relevant findings are presented.

In addition to participating in the interview, the parents were all asked to complete the Cornell Medical Index at the time of the interview, and parent-attitude questionnaires were sent out later. Details of these are provided later in the book.

Arrangement of the survey records

Family composition, household composition, other significant adults.

Description of housing type and amenities, standard of equipment and care.

Description of interview.

The parents' childhoods and personalities – childhood, education, occupational history, service record, personality and interests, occupation of grandparents.

Summary of consultation record in general practice.

Description of the marriage.

Ratings of the marital relationship–discrepancies, decision-making, social activities, overall rating.

Child's history – pregnancy, infancy, physical handicaps, recurrent complaints, hospital admissions, other separations, schooling history, trouble with authority.

Macfarlane ratings (descriptions of children's personality and symptoms).

Child's social participation, attitude to school.

Summary of school report.

Summary of general practice consultations on the child.

State of siblings not included in the survey.

Account of child-rearing attitudes.

Child-rearing attitude scales.

The family as a unit – external relationships, social participation, management, general conclusions.

Joint summary made after assembly of all the above data.

CHAPTER 2

The Social Circumstances and Characteristics of the Population

> It is the disaster of London, as to the beauty of its figure, that
> it is stretched out in buildings, just as the pleasure of every
> builder, or undertaker of buildings, and as the convenience of
> the people directs, whether for trade or otherwise; and this
> has spread the face of it in a most straggling, confus'd
> manner, out of all shape, uncompact, and unequal . . .
>
> Daniel Defoe, *A tour through England and Wales*

The population from which the 112 families were drawn consisted of patients registered on my National Health Service list. The practice is in a working-class London borough, and dates back to before the Lloyd George Act of 1911, my own predecessor having taken over from the original doctor in 1919. Shortly after I entered the practice in 1952 the building, which had originally housed the doctor's family as well as the two practice rooms, was converted with the help of a group practice loan, and an initial partnership of three doctors, later increased to four, was formed. By 1959, when the family survey started, my patients were divided fairly equally into those inherited from my predecessor and those recruited in the intervening years.

Every family in this registered population in which there was at least one child of primary school age (born during the years 1949–55), and one parent registered, was selected. From this group those known to be in Social Classes I and II were excluded, because this group was too small to offer a possibility of investigating class differences and also because it contained a large proportion of personal friends; in fact a small number of Class I and II families, mostly small traders, was included. A further one or two families were excluded because of language problems, or because they were known to be on the verge of rehousing outside the area, and one family where the child had a potentially fatal illness was not included. The remainder, numbering

121 families, were approached and 112 co-operated. This class selection, and the small distance of most of the patients' homes from the practice centre had the effect of producing a population relatively homogeneous in its social characteristics. As our main interest was in intrafamilial processes this was an advantage.

As mentioned, the practice is situated in an old London working-class industrial borough, with industry and housing intermingled, engineering and the railways providing the main local employment. The population of the borough had been falling for some years before the war and the trend has continued. The general standard of housing is still poor, but seldom appalling, a typical home being a part of a large mid-Victorian terrace house, with a minority of families in self-contained old houses or (increasingly) council flats. As the parents had all been married for six or more years (apart from two remarriages), most had acquired some degree of independence in their housing, although half the sample had started their married lives in the home of one or other grandparent, and a further thirteen in furnished rooms. Housing difficulties and worries still loomed large in the lives of many, in terms both of the physical inconvenience of many of the dwellings, and of the lack of freedom and the irritations of shared accommodation, and the feeling of interference from relatives. The standard of housing amenity was rated according to the scale reproduced at the end of this chapter, in which points were awarded for the degree of overcrowding, the sleeping arrangements, and for the possession of separate bathroom, kitchen, and W.C. On this scale there are four grades: good, fair, poor, and very poor. Of the 99 married couples, 38 had good homes, 35 fair, 17 poor, and 9 very poor homes; of the families with one parent, only one had good and two had fair accommodation, five being poorly and five very poorly housed. Examples of these grades are as follows:

1. *Good housing:* A family with three children aged between 10 and 17 living in a self-contained borough council conversion consisting of five rooms with their own bathroom, kitchen/dining-room, and indoor W.C. Two boys share a bedroom in single beds and the girl has a room of her own. Spacious rooms with large windows.
2. *Fair housing:* A family with single parent (mother) and five children aged between 3 and 13. A self-contained borough

25

council flat in a small block built since the war and consisting of four rooms including a kitchen/living-room, a bathroom, and an indoor W.C. The youngest daughter shared the mother's bed, and the two other bedrooms each contained two of the boys.

3. *Poor housing:* A family with three children, aged 8 and 14, living in a self-contained flat in a private house. There are two rooms, a kitchen, an indoor W.C., but no bath. The parents sleep in one room and the children share the other.

4. *Very poor housing:* A family with five children aged between 2 and 10, inhabiting a non-self-contained flat consisting of two rooms, their own kitchen, with an indoor W.C. shared with four others. Children and parents all share one bedroom, two girls sharing one bed and the two boys another, one boy having his own bed. No bathroom.

On the whole, the standard of equipment of the families was better than the standard of their housing. An index of possessions, in which different articles were allotted from one to three points, was drawn up, and this is reproduced in an appendix at the end of this chapter. *Table 1* gives the distribution of the population according to the

TABLE 1 'POSSESSIONS RATING' OF 112 FAMILIES

Home equipped	99 Couples	13 Single parents
Very well	28	0
Well	29	2
Adequately	22	5
Poorly	20	6

possessions rating. For example, to be classified as very well equipped a family might have a car, telephone, refrigerator, washing machine, and television, while to be classified as poorly equipped they would have no more than a washing machine or television and a vacuum cleaner. As with housing standards, the poorer status of families with one parent is evident. This is an effect of the fact that 11 of the 13 such families are headed by the mother alone, and the economic problems of these families are underlined by the figures for income levels given in *Table 2*. Income levels for the families were calculated as the joint income of both parents less tax and insurance but not

TABLE 2   FAMILY INCOME OF 112 FAMILIES

Family weekly income	99 Couples	13 Single parents
Under £10	0	7
£10–14	18	3
£15–19	40	2
£20 or more	36	1
Not recorded	5	0

including family allowances. Women made a significant contribution to family income in a large proportion of the families, since, of the 99 married couples, the women were in full time work (i.e. more than 26 hours per week) in 27, and in part time work in 32. The distribution of the population by social class according to the Registrar General's classification is given in *Table 3*, which also records the number of

TABLE 3   SOCIAL CLASS OF 99 COUPLES RELATED TO OTHER
SOCIAL INDICES

Social class	Number	Wives at work (whole or part time)		Income of £20 or more		Home very well equipped	
		No.	%	No.	%	No.	%
I or II	13	4	31	9	70	7	54
III	63	40	64	25	40	14	22
IV or V	23	15	65	7	30	7	30
Total	99	59	60	41	41	28	28

wives working, and the income and the possessions rating according to class. Class gradients are not marked, but it should be recalled that many of those in Classes I and II were in fact local small traders, differing little from their employed neighbours, and it should be noted that only four families were in Social Class V. Social class shift was assessed in the case of the fathers by comparing their occupational status with that of their fathers, and in the case of women by comparing the occupational status of their husbands with that of their fathers. About one quarter of the men showed upward mobility, and one quarter downward mobility, and a similar proportion of the women showed social class shifts by marriage. However, in view of the relatively small class differences in status and income level within this population the significance of this shift is uncertain.

In 78 of the 99 now-married couples, at least one partner was locally bred. In 44 instances both husband and wife were born in the borough, and in a further 13 both were born in London. Only 16 couples were both born outside London, most of these being Irish. In view of this it is not surprising to find a high degree of contact with the extended family. Classification of the population according to their contact with the grandparents is given in *Table 4*. It is seen that

TABLE 4 FREQUENCY OF CONTACT WITH OWN PARENTS OF 99 COUPLES

Contact with own parents	Number	Virtu- ally daily	Less than daily, more than weekly	Less than weekly, more than monthly	Less than monthly, more than yearly	Seldom or never
Fathers	99	13	31	12	8	35
Mothers	99	20	28	3	14	34

one in five of the mothers and one in seven of the fathers had virtually daily contact with their own parents, and that the proportion seeing their parents at least weekly was nearly half for both mothers and fathers. If contact with siblings is included, then only one in three of the mothers had infrequent contact with her family (i.e. less than monthly), the proportion being only slightly higher in the case of the fathers. These figures are of the same order as those described by Young and Willmott (1962) in Bethnal Green. The frequency of contact is somewhat lower for the men than for the women, which is also in keeping with their findings. It is, of course, more common for regular exchange of services to occur between mother and daughter, whereas the husband's visit to his parents is more likely to be a purely social engagement. The actual content of the relationship of the parents with their own parents varied a great deal: in many cases there was an element of dependence upon the grandparents both for moral support and for practical help; in other cases there was the reverse situation, with some dependence on the part of the older generation. Not infrequently these relationships were a source of tension and conflict. The origins of neurosis are often found in the relationship with the parents in childhood; it is clearly important to recognize that parents continue to play an important role for many adults, quite apart from their 'internalized' one.

Apart from contact with the extended family and casual gossiping with neighbours at the street corner, the parents of most families remained relatively isolated from their society. The only local organizations to attract much support were the tenants' associations which, at the time of the survey, were involved in agitation over rent issues. These bodies also provided one of the few regular social activities in the neighbourhood. A classification of the families was made on the basis of the extent of the parents' social contacts; this classification is given below with the numbers classified in each category.

Parents' social participation scale

1. *Isolated families* (Six couples and two single-parent families): In these families there is no contact with or support from either the extended family or from friends; there may be some 'interference' from outside sources which is resented: these families appear to be potentially dependent but without appropriate support.
2. *Dependent families* (23 couples and five single-parent families): In these, relationships are confined to the extended family or perhaps one or two friends, but are characterized by dependence and immaturity. Included in this group are some dependent upon social agencies.
3. *Partially integrated families* (51 couples and five single-parent families): In these families there are relationships with the extended family or some friends; wider contacts may occur but are confined to one parent only.
4. *Integrated families* (Seven couples and one single-parent family): In these families both parents have satisfactory relationships outside the home with a reasonable social circle.
5. *Socially oriented families* (Ten couples): These have, in addition to the features of the integrated families, some active participation by one or both parents in some community activity, i.e. trade union work, youth work, etc.
6. *Socially active families* (Two families): In these, in addition to the features of the two previous groups, one or both parents are office holders in some community body.

Further light upon the integration of the couples with the local social life is provided by the classification of social activity, defined as more or less organized outings to dances, cinemas, or other recreational activities. Of the 99 married couples, 48 never participated in this type of activity together, and 56 of the wives and 32 of the husbands never had any independent social activity.

In general, therefore, one may say that the survey families were characterized by a high degree of continued contact with their own extended families, and with a low degree of contact or participation in other social activities. This somewhat isolated picture must be complemented by noting that a large proportion of the couples obviously gained considerable reward from their homes, and had much pride and satisfaction in them. If one sometimes felt that the pattern of family life was rather limited, one had to remember that poverty, physical discomfort, and lack of privacy characterized the childhood homes of a large proportion of the parents; to have provided a better home for their own children was no mean achievement, and was a source of great satisfaction.

Having outlined the social characteristics of the population, we must now consider how far it is permissible to generalize from the findings – that is to say, to ask how typical this population may be. Any study of a limited population is bound, to some extent, to be applicable only to the population studied. Factors that could lead to bias in our population, apart from the social and geographical features outlined above, could include selection by virtue of being registered on one doctor's list. It is certain that some selective recruitment of doctors by patients occurs, and it is possible that my interest in psychiatry might have attracted an undue proportion of emotionally disturbed patients. However, I believe this process to be relatively uncommon. The inclusion in the design of the study of a certain number of standard instruments permitted us to compare our population with larger samples similarly tested. In respect of neuroticism we have, for most of the parents, scores on the Cornell Medical Index (C.M.I.) which are reported fully later in the book, and equivalent figures are now obtainable from two other English populations. One of these is a practice in Beckenham (Brown and Fry, 1962) and the other is a study of a number of practices (including my own and my partners') made by the Nuffield Research Unit of the Institute of Psychiatry (B. Cooper, personal communication). *Table 5* shows that

Social Circumstances and Characteristics of the Population

Sex	Population	Sample size	C.M.I. Score 30 or more[1]	
			No.	%
Male	Survey population	101	14	14
	Fry's practices (aged 20–60)	76	9	12
	Cooper's survey (aged 25–44)	376	58	15
Female	Survey population	110	38	35
	Fry's practices (aged 20–60)	94	24	26
	Cooper's survey (aged 25–44)	505	196	39

[1]In the case of the Survey population scoring 31 or more.

the distribution of C.M.I. scores for the parents in the survey population was similar to that in the other populations investigated.

Other standard tests administered to our survey population included parental attitude inventories. In the case of the mothers' inventory, the mean scores for Acceptance and Domination recorded by our mothers were within the range found by A. N. Oppenheim in testing a large representative sample (personal communication). In the case of the fathers, the mean Domination scores were lower than those recorded on a South London population of rather lower social class composition. In general, therefore, it would seem that the survey population can probably be taken as reasonably representative of the London middle working class.

APPENDIX TO CHAPTER 2

Housing amenity scale

Amenity	Features	Score
Bathroom:	Own	2
	Shared	1
Kitchen:	Own in separate room	1
W.C.:	Own W.C.	1
	Indoors	1
Parents' bedroom:	No children	2
	Children under 5 only	1
Children's bedroom:	At least one child has own bedroom	2
	Fewer than 4 children share bedroom in separate beds	1
Crowding index:	Number of rooms (excluding kitchen, W.C.) divided by number in household: Index of 0·5–1	2
	1·0–1·5	4
	1·5+	6

Total scores: 0–4 Very poor; 5–7 Poor; 8–10 Fair; 11–16 Good.

Possessions index

Possession	Score
Telephone	3
Motor-cycle	2
Car	3
Other special equipment	2
Radiogram	1
Refrigerator	2
Vacuum cleaner	1
Washing machine	2
TV	1
Tape recorder	2

Total scores: 11+ Very well equipped; 8–10 Well equipped;
4–7 Adequately equipped; 0–3 Poorly equipped.

CHAPTER 3

The Parents' Childhoods

There are no memories more precious than those of one's
early childhood in one's own home, and that is almost
always so, if there is any love and harmony in the family at
all. Indeed precious memories may be retained even from a
bad home so long as your heart is capable of finding anything
precious.

Father Zossima in *The Brothers Karamazov*
by Feodor Dostoyevsky (translated by David Magarshak)

The parents of the 112 families studied (101 men and 110 women)
were aged between the mid-twenties and mid-fifties at the time of the
survey, with a median age in the mid-thirties (see *Table 6*). Most of

TABLE 6   AGE DISTRIBUTION OF PARENTS

Age	Fathers	Mothers
Under 25	0	1
25–34	33	53
35–44	50	46
45 or more	18	10
Total	101	110

the parents were therefore born around the time of the economic
depression, and had their schooling or their first jobs interrupted by
the war. A number of them were old enough to have served in the
armed forces during the war. In recording their childhoods, it soon
became clear that adversity of one sort or another was more common
than not: few could look back upon a childhood undisturbed by
hardship or unhappiness. It also became clear that hardship and unhappiness did not necessarily go together: phrases such as 'Dad was

C

often out of work and we had a rough time, but Mum was a real brick – we made our own amusements in those days', suggest a picture of successful family functioning despite adversity. Some, on the other hand, would report to the effect that 'We never lacked for nothing, but Mum was always on at Dad and on at us – no wonder the old man spent the weekends at the pub; somehow there was no love in her.' We developed a classification of childhood experience which concentrated upon the emotional tone of the home. This classification is reproduced below, the number of individuals in each category being recorded, and a case history chosen at random being provided to illustrate each category. Obviously these reports are highly subjective and unverifiable, and the amount of detail provided varied greatly between different informants. In most cases, however, the talk was clearly too spontaneous, and often too charged with emotion, for any conscious deception to be operating. However, in using the evidence of the recollection of childhood experience one must be aware of the limitations, even though it is our impression from the detail provided and from those cases where we had more than one parent from the same family in our survey that accuracy was in fact high. It would be dangerous to draw firm conclusions about the aetiology of adult neurosis from such data, and this reservation must be borne in mind when considering the figures provided later in the book which show associations between recalled childhood factors and current adjustment and behaviour. Having said this, it may be pointed out that in fact the child's perception of his family, and the adult's recollection of his childhood, are quite possibly of greater relevance to his emotional health than is the 'objective reality' to which he was exposed. This may perhaps be illustrated by quoting the descriptions of childhood given by three parents who were siblings. The eldest, James, said that he had only good memories of childhood: there was 'nothing to be remembered with hate'; they had a reasonable standard of living, with good holidays, and the father never hit any of the children because 'he didn't need to – if he called once we were there'. At the interview he said that he did recall an occasion when the younger sister, Jean, had been struck by the father and how upset the father had been. However, the second member of the family, Jean, who was two years younger, recalled being 'petrified' of the father until her late teens. She described him as having had a filthy temper, and said that when in a temper he would clout blindly. He always insisted that what he said was done, and as she was something of a rebel she got a good deal more punishment from him than did her siblings. Her mother would occasionally try to protect or defend her. She was evacuated from home at the age of eleven. Her sister Doris, six years younger, described her childhood as happy. She was away with Jean from the age of six to twelve during the war, and she recalled this period as being extremely happy and she was reluctant to return home. Doris's childhood was rated emotionally secure as was her brother's, but Jean's was rated as showing minor emotional disturbance. This would seem to be a case in which possibly her recollection had exaggerated a situation in which she, by temperament, provoked a different response from her father, and therefore did in fact experience him in a different way.

The classification of childhood experience contains six categories, of which 1–3 are classified as emotionally secure and 4–6 as emotionally disturbed. Details of the classification, with examples selected from the category at random, are provided as follows:

Category 1, no adverse experience (41 fathers and 24 mothers): Mr Brown, aged 35 at the time of the interview, was the fourth of five children born in a small country town. He reported that his childhood was the happiest time of his life. It was a hard life in the country and he was frequently belted by the parents, but 'that was just their way'. All the children in the family were treated alike, and there was a strong bond between them.

Category 2, poverty or ill health but, in other respects, emotionally secure (13 men and 14 women): Mr Green, aged 50 at the time of the interview, was the eldest of the three surviving children. He was brought up in comfortable circumstances and remembers his home as being happy in childhood, although later as an adolescent he rebelled against his father. His mother, however, was incapacitated, and had to run her household from a wheelchair. He spent a period of two months away from home in an isolation hospital but does not remember this as being an unhappy experience.

Category 3, loss of one or both parents, but in other respects emotionally secure (Nine men and seven women): In this group the lost parent was adequately substituted for by the remaining parent or by a stable and continuing alternative figure, and there was no other emotional disturbance. An example is provided by Mrs Black, who was 42 at the time of the survey interview. She was the youngest of seven children and 'had a very happy childhood with lots of pets'. She was spoilt by her father although he was strict. Her mother died when she was ten. She had been very good-natured and affectionate, and Mrs Black was very upset at her death and still missed her, often thinking 'how dreadful it was to be left without a mother so young'. The rest of the family helped run the house until her father's remarriage four years later. The stepmother was 'quite nice', but Mrs Black was unable to form any close attachment to her. However, she is classified in this category in view of the uninterrupted good relationship with her father.

Category 4, an intact home with minor emotional disturbance (16 men and 34 women): Minor disturbance is characterized as frequent verbal quarrelling between parents, or inadequate affection from the parents, or emotional instability in one parent; or harshness, or differentiation of the individual from his or her siblings. An example is provided by Mrs White, who was the only girl in a large family. Throughout her childhood her mother was ill and often bedridden, and the girl missed much schooling by being kept at home to help in the house. She felt picked upon by her mother, who was thought to have resented the fact that she (Mrs White) was a girl. She had a rather better relationship with her father, but he also was ill and frequently unemployed.

Category 5, intact home but with major emotional disturbance (11 men and 12 women): Under major disturbance we include physically violent quarrelling between the parents or physical ill-treatment of the child, or major mental illness or problem drinking in one parent, or other major emotional deprivation. Mrs Gray was the younger of two children. She remembered being very unsure of herself as a child, her mother being 'a hard and violent woman with no time for the children', and the girl was in fact physically neglected, on one occasion losing a large amount of her hair due to an untreated lice-infested and secondarily infected scalp. This, and being bombed out, interrupted her education. Her father was a weak man dominated by the mother.

Category 6, loss of one or both parents in addition to emotional disturbance of the types described in Categories 4 and 5 (11 men and 19 women): An example is provided by Mr Rose, in his forties at the time of interview. He was the youngest of four children, his mother died while bearing him, and he was brought up by a stepmother. He was rather reticent about his childhood, but mentioned a lot of quarrelling, though no physical violence. He described his stepmother as 'rather cool, but about average for a stepmother'.

It is notable that women report a much higher rate of minor emotional disturbance than do men. This may reflect a difference in recall or different standards for emotional security between women and men. It is also probable that girls are more exposed to the stresses of disturbance in a family than are boys.

The other main childhood factor recorded was the educational level achieved. This was classified into three levels:

1. Those who left school at or before 15 and had no further training (66 men and 74 women).
2. Those who remained at school beyond 15 or took some alternative trades training or apprenticeship, or attended night school (30 men and 24 women).
3. A small group who went further than this, taking an examination more or less equivalent to the General Certificate of Education (5 men and 12 women).

CHAPTER 4

Neurosis in the Parents and its
Relation to Childhood and Social Factors

> One writes of scars healed, a loose parallel to the pathology of
> the skin, but there is no such thing in the life of an individual.
> There are open wounds, shrunk sometimes to the size of a
> pin-prick, but wounds still. The marks of suffering are more
> comparable to the loss of a finger, or of the sight of an eye.
> We may not miss them, either, for one minute in a year, but
> if we should there is nothing to be done about it.
>
> F. Scott Fitzgerald, *Tender is the night*

Neurosis in the parents was assessed by two methods: the first by examination of my own routine practice consultation records, and the second the Cornell Medical Index, which was completed by nearly all the parents. Consultation records were analysed for the previous five years, and any patient who had presented in that time with neurotic symptoms (but not with psychosomatic symptoms alone) was classified as neurotic. The C.M.I. has by now been widely used and appears to be an instrument of reasonable validity, although no formal validation studies have been carried out. It consists of 175 questions concerning symptoms, divided into an organic section (A–L) and a psychiatric section (M–R). To each question the respondent answers by ringing Yes or No. For the purposes of measuring neuroticism, a total Yes score, plus the number of comments and corrections, provides a single score which seems as capable as many more refined methods of distinguishing neurotics from non-neurotics. High score levels have been shown to be more common in neurotics than in normals among out-patient attenders (Culpan *et al.*, 1960; Brodman *et al.*, 1949, 1951, 1952), to be associated with poorer army service records (Brodman *et al.*, 1954) and to be related to a general practice diagnosis of neurosis (Brown and Fry, 1962).

In the study of part of the survey population we found that a diagnosis from my records was significantly associated with a high C.M.I. score, though there were some patients who had consulted who scored relatively low, and a number of high scorers who had not consulted; in nearly all the latter group Miss Hamilton's interview gave confirmatory evidence of neurosis (Ryle and Hamilton, 1962). The Yes responses in the 'organic' section (A–L) of the C.M.I. were shown in women to consist largely of symptoms of a functional type; this was not apparent in the case of the men (Hamilton *et al.*, 1962). For most statistical calculations we have used the C.M.I. score as a single indicator of neurosis, taking a score of 31 or more as definitely neurotic, and one of 16–30 as moderately so. For some group comparisons the mean C.M.I. scores have been used. A few parents, however, did not complete the Cornell Medical Index: in some calculations this group was excluded, but for other purposes a classification into non-neurotic and neurotic by minimal criteria was used, individuals with 'minimal neurosis' being those with a score of 16 or more on the C.M.I. or with a psychiatric consultation over the previous five years.

Tables 7 and *8* demonstrate the association between childhood experience and neurosis, as measured by the C.M.I. score and by minimal criteria. It is seen that those in the emotionally secure childhood categories were less often neurotic than those in the emotionally disturbed ones, the difference in rates being significant at the 10 per cent level only, except in the case of minimal neurosis in women ($p < 0.01$). The lower number of men than of women with high C.M.I.

TABLE 7   RELATIONSHIP BETWEEN CHILDHOOD EXPERIENCE
AND NEUROSIS (110 MOTHERS)

Childhood experience category	Number	No. with minimal neurosis	No. with[1] C.M.I. of 31 or more	Mean C.M.I.[2]
Secure	45	26	11	23·5
Disturbed	65	56	27	35·7
Whole population	110	82	38	31·1

[1]A disturbed childhood is related significantly to the presence of minimal neurosis ($\chi^2 = 9.7$, $p < 0.01$) and to a C.M.I. score of 31+ at the 10 per cent level ($\chi^2 = 2.7$).
[2]C.M.I. completed by 106.

TABLE 8   RELATIONSHIP BETWEEN CHILDHOOD EXPERIENCE
AND NEUROSIS (101 FATHERS)

Childhood experience category	Number	No. with minimal neurosis	No. with C.M.I. of 31 or more[1]	Mean C.M.I.[2]
Secure	63	27	5	15·3
Disturbed	38	24	9	22·1
Whole population	101	51	14	17·9

[1]A disturbed childhood is related at the 10 per cent level of significance to the presence of minimal neurosis ($\chi^2 = 3·1$) and to a C.M.I. score of 31+ ($\chi^2 = 3·7$).
[2]C.M.I. completed by 98.

scores (found in all studies) may in part reflect the items included in the index; however, it is in line with the figures for consultation rates for neurosis from my own and other general practice studies (Ryle, 1960; Kessel and Shepherd, 1962).

The association demonstrated between recalled childhood experience and adult neuroticism is, at first glance, likely to be a causal one, and is in accordance with the findings of the few other workers who have reported similar studies (e.g. Ingham, 1949, and Petursson, 1961). However, the reservation made earlier about retrospective evidence must be borne in mind. It could be argued that neuroticism is an inherited tendency manifested by both parents and children, or that neurotics magnify in recollection the hardships of their childhoods. While I doubt whether either of these explanations accounts for the whole association, neither can be ruled out on the evidence provided.

Many other aspects of the parents' lives, which have already been discussed in outline, might be expected to bear some relationship to their liability to neurosis. Aspects that concern the relationship between the parents are discussed, together with other factors connected with the marriages, in the next chapter. Of the remaining social factors, none in fact showed any significant association with neuroticism. Frequent job changes (other than those involving promotion) were slightly more common amongst neurotic men, but not significantly so. Women at work were neither more nor less neurotic than those who were whole-time housewives. Social class, according to the Registrar

General's classification, showed no significant association with neuroticism, nor did social mobility; but the limitations of this rather crude classification, and the relative homogeneity of our population, must be borne in mind. Such tendencies as were apparent were in fact in the direction of a lower rate of neurosis in the lower social classes and in those downwardly mobile. Social aspirations for house ownership were unrelated to neuroticism, but strong educational aspirations for the children, expressed in a marked desire for them to pass the 11 plus or in an intention to pay for private education, were more often expressed by neurotic women. This is probably a reflection of over-involvement rather than of a more general social attitude.

The rate of neurosis (by minimal criteria or by a C.M.I. score of 31 +) was rather higher in the wives of couples where one or both were immigrants to London, than in those where both were locally born; there was no difference in the case of the men. This difference was not significant, and was probably associated with the higher proportion in the immigrant group reporting adverse childhood experience. The same comment applies to the relationship which was found to exist between the frequency of contact with the extended families and neurosis: the rate of neurosis in both men and women was somewhat higher in the group who had little or no contact with the extended family, but once again, the rate of adverse childhood experience in this group was higher than in those with more contact; this probably reflects the fact that individuals are more likely to lose contact with their family where the home has been an unhappy one. The numbers recorded as having had psychiatric treatment in the practice, and the numbers given more prolonged treatment or referred for hospital treatment, did not differ significantly between those with frequent and those with infrequent or no contact with the extended family, such differences as there were being in the direction of more consultation and referral in those with frequent family contact.

Epidemiological medicine, with its roots in public health, has been largely preoccupied with major social factors such as social class, and this preoccupation has been echoed in the classics of social psychiatry (e.g. Faris and Dunham, 1939; Hare, 1956; Hollingshead and Redlich, 1958; Ødegaard, 1945, 1956; Norris, 1959).

Most of this work has been concerned with the psychoses, and studies of the association of neurosis with social factors have been less frequent and less fertile. It remains a task of considerable size to devise definitions and criteria of neurosis that can be applied equally in different social groups; and even were this task surmounted, the relationship between major social factors and neurosis is likely to be a tenuous one with a large number of intervening variables. This being so, the neglect of family and small group studies of neurosis, particularly this side of the Atlantic, is surprising. Being based upon a relatively homogeneous population, our study was not designed primarily to assess social factors. It is of interest that the few trends suggesting possible association between neurosis, and the social variables measured could be explained largely in terms of the one clearly relevant variable, namely the individual's recollection of the emotional tone of his childhood home. This, and the following chapters, may serve to underline the suggestion that the most productive focus for research into neurosis is likely to be the family.

Recalling their childhood was obviously a moving experience for many of the informants, and several commented on how the presentation of their stories had served to 'put things into perspective'. This perspective, no doubt, was in part that imposed by the frame of reference of our research and by Miss Hamilton's role as social worker. An inquiry using more structured techniques would have been easier to record and rate, but it would not have tapped the same fund of recollection and of feeling, and it would have been correspondingly less relevant as a contribution to an understanding of the family.

CHAPTER 5

The Parents' Marriages

That's Venus' method. According to whim
She puts bodies and minds to work her brass yoke
In incongruous pairs – and enjoys the bad joke.
Horace, *Odes* (translated by James Michie)

Marriage is the central relationship of most adults in our society. It is a relationship of significance in many different areas of life, within which many different facets of individual personality are expressed. No investigation can hope to take full account of its complexity: to make any investigation and report manageable, some splitting up of the functions of the marriage relationship must be carried out, even though in reality the personalities of the individuals and the form of the relationship are closely interrelated. A major division into two aspects can be made as follows: (a) marriage as the fundamental relationship of the family, with its task as the socialization of children – the subject matter of later chapters; and (b) marriage as a relationship between two adults, having both economic and emotional functions – the subject matter of the present chapter.

In the following account of the marriages in our population a number of discrete aspects of the relationship are discussed – relating to the courtship history, to the economic roles of the husbands and wives, to some social characteristics of the couples, and, tentatively, to patterns of interaction. Presented in this way, however, the picture might well prove too confusing and fragmented to be of interest. Consequently, many of the individual descriptive measures have been related to a more general assessment of the extent to which the marriage appears to have fulfilled its overall social and emotional function. This assessment was made against a five-point rating scale, described below. Some of these individual measures are illustrated by extracts from case histories, which also offer an impression of the type of data which was obtained at the survey interviews and from routine practice records. At the end of the chapter, certain aspects of the marital relationship are related to the presence or absence of neurosis in the marital partners.

THE MARITAL RATING

The overall assessment of the marriage relationship was made against the following five-point scale (stable, non-legal unions being counted as marriage):

1. *Good adjustment* – warm, positive feeling, shared interests and activities.
2. *Adequate adjustment* – willing and able to discuss differences.
3. *Stresses contained within the marriage.*
4. *Open conflict* – marriage sustained by social pressure or abnormal attitudes.
5. *Broken marriage* (includes never established).

Clearly, the wording of this scale conveys some value judgement as to what constitutes a good marriage, in particular placing emphasis upon the emotional aspects of the relationship; this was deliberate as this would seem to be the one of most relevance to psychiatry. To reduce the dangers of subjectivity in making this rating, each couple in the population was rated against the scale by two observers: Miss Hamilton, on the basis of her survey interview; and myself, independently, on the basis of my routine contacts over the years with the family. The reliability of my rating was clearly variable, depending upon the length and degree of contact – more detailed information being available for those couples who had consulted with problems in their marriage relationship, and no rating being made on a small proportion of the couples. Even given two observers, however, the possibility of bias remained in that the assumptions held by Miss Hamilton and myself were similar in most respects and might, for example, have reflected class preconceptions. As an additional measure, therefore, the couple at interview were asked to say how they felt their marriage compared with that of their contemporaries, the replies being recorded verbatim. Where one or both indicated a definite opinion that their marriage was either more or less successful than average, this was recorded. The distribution of the 99 couples by Miss Hamilton's rating, and the comparative judgements of myself and of the couple concerned, are recorded in *Table 9*. This table,

TABLE 9 RELATIONSHIP BETWEEN THE P.S.W. MARITAL RATING, THE G.P.'S INDEPENDENT RATING, AND THE COUPLE'S OWN ASSESSMENT

Marital rating (P.S.W.)	Number	G.P. rated		Couple rated	
		Higher[1]	Lower[1]	Above average	Below average
1	15	0	12	14	0
2	39	4	4	30	0
3	37	19	1	15	2
4	8	2	0	0	6
Total	99	25	17	59	8

[1]In all cases by one point only.

while showing a fairly high proportion where there was a discrepancy of one point between Miss Hamilton and myself, may, I believe, be taken as showing reasonable agreement, and as suggesting that the criteria of bad adjustment applied in our rating do not differ markedly from the criteria used by the couples themselves. As Miss Hamilton's rating was in most instances based upon fuller evidence than my own, her classification has been adopted in the tables which follow.

The majority of the features being assessed in this chapter refer to factors which have not necessarily any direct bearing upon the marital rating. In these tables, therefore, tests of statistical significance (χ^2 test using Yates's correction) are provided for any associations found between the feature and the marital rating. The first two factors, however, relate to functions of central importance to the marriage relationship, and the information upon which these ratings was based clearly played a large part in determining the overall rating. Tests of significance would be inappropriate here.

COMMUNICATION

The ability of a husband and wife to communicate their ideas and feelings to each other was rated against the following scale:

1. *Good:* able to express feelings openly and directly; to resolve differences successfully, even if after arguments, without the need for either to swallow resentment or to act out to achieve their objective; both able to compromise.
2. *Fair:* able to communicate in many areas, but there are some in which one or other cannot express feelings due either to his or her own difficulties or to the spouse's anticipated response; include under this heading the habitual use of 'hurt' responses.
3. *Poor:* inability or refusal to communicate feelings or needs; non-problem-solving types of protest activity; extreme rigidity or emotional distance ruling out any possibility of compromise; include here deliberate exclusion or deception.

This rating was made jointly by myself and Miss Hamilton on the basis of her interview records; it paralleled closely the overall marital rating. An example of a couple rated as 'poor' on this scale is given in the following description.

Mr and Mrs Home were interviewed together for most of the time, although one interview was with the mother alone. In describing the couple, both the interview material and my own records showed evidence that the mother was an inhibited, somewhat obsessional, personality, and the father a rather dominant and cold one. Miss Hamilton's record, which described their disagreements and solution of differences, read as follows: 'There were quite severe rows in the early days of the marriage, as father was out too often visiting the dog tracks, gambling, etc. Mother felt he was getting into bad company. Now there are very few quarrels, because "one can't argue with him". The father, however, can be outspoken if things don't please him, whereas the mother tends to keep her feelings and opinions to herself lest she be accused of nagging. They never disagree over money, but they may do over the children: for example the father often takes the mother to task for shouting at them. They can't easily talk things out together as the father tends to make a joke about mother's complaints or opinions or else walks out, whereas mother tends to swallow her dissatisfactions with her husband for the sake of peace. The mother describes the father as hard, "like the rest of his family". He never shows sympathy, and cannot show feelings of any sort. She feels hurt that he is never able to buy her a present himself, although he may give her money to go out and buy one for herself "a thing he does ungraciously and infrequently".'

SEXUAL ADJUSTMENT

Understandably, not all couples were willing or able to give information about their sexual adjustment. No information was obtained, in fact, in one quarter of the sample. Of the remainder, about one half had a satisfactory relationship and the other half a poor one (see *Table 10* for the scale and distribution).

TABLE 10   RELATIONSHIP OF MARITAL RATING TO SEXUAL ADJUSTMENT RATING

Sexual adjustment	Number	Marital rating			
		1	2	3	4
Mutually satisfactory	18	5	11	2	0
Minor disparity, well tolerated	17	3	9	4	1
Total 'satisfactory'	35	8	20	6	1
Frequent rejection or reluctance or *coitus interruptus*	30	1	8	15	6
Absent, infrequent, or always resented	7	0	2	5	0
Total 'poor'	37	1	10	20	6
Not known	27	6	9	11	1
Total	99	15	39	37	8

Not surprisingly, a good rating for sexual adjustment parallels fairly closely the general marital rating. Couples not providing information showed the same distribution on the marital rating as did the remainder of the population; hence it seems likely that the proportion with satisfactory sexual adjustment is a reasonably representative one. It should, however, be noted that by no means all of those rated as poor expressed active dissatisfaction. Some, especially among the men, were satisfied with *coitus interruptus*, and some, particularly among the women, seemed to accept the non-achievement – or, more often, the extinction – of a sexual basis for their relationship as a part of the natural order of things. On the other hand, some of the wives

47

in the couples rated 2 on the scale seemed to be providing a willing service rather than experiencing any positive satisfaction.

THE ANTECEDENTS AND ORIGINS OF THE COUPLE RELATED TO THEIR MARITAL ADJUSTMENT

The state of a marriage at a given time reflects both the personalities and previous experiences of the couple and the effect of the inter-action between them. In this section, certain factors relating to the early life and the courtship of the couple will be described in relation to their current marital rating. It should be recalled at this point that, apart from two remarriages, the couples had all been married or cohabiting for at least six years at the time of the interview.

(a) Childhood experience

The criteria for the classification of childhood experience into adverse or secure have already been described in Chapter 4. The classification of the couples according to the childhood experience of each is give in *Table 11*. It is noteworthy that there is no tendency for husband and wife to come from similarly rated childhood backgrounds. Couples where both had experienced secure childhoods had better rated marriages than the rest, though this association is significant at the 10 per cent level only ($\chi^2 = 3.5$).

TABLE 11 RELATIONSHIP OF MARITAL RATING TO CLASSIFICATION OF THE CHILDHOOD EXPERIENCE OF THE COUPLE

Childhood experience			Marital rating			
Father	Mother	Number	1	2	3	4
Secure	Secure	28	6	14	8	0
Secure	Disturbed	34	4	12	14	4
Disturbed	Secure	14	3	4	5	2
Disturbed	Disturbed	23	2	9	10	2

(b) Age at marriage and premarital conception

In nearly one quarter of all marriages the first child had been con-ceived before marriage, this proportion rising steeply with decrease in age, as is apparent from *Table 12*. Not all of these marriages were forced by social pressure, for, in some instances, conception was deliberately used as a means of overcoming parental opposition to the marriage. In *Table 12* it is seen that the more youthful marriages, despite their much higher rate of premarital conception, receive better ratings than do the later ones – an association which is quite insignificant but which at least throws doubt upon the contrary assumption that age and maturity enable a wiser choice of marriage partner to be made. One must add that those couples who conceive premaritally and subsequently marry are obviously not a random sample of all extramarital conceptions.

TABLE 12 RELATIONSHIP OF MARITAL RATING TO
AGE AT MARRIAGE AND TO PREMARITAL CONCEPTION

Age of youngest at marriage	*Number*	*Premarital conception*	*Marital rating*			
			1	*2*	*3*	*4*
Under 18	15	11	2 (2)	8 (5)	4 (4)	1
18–21	43	10	8 (1)	17 (6)	18 (3)	2
22–25	28	1	3	9	13	3 (1)
26–30	10	0	1	4	4	1
31 or more	3	1	1 (1)	1	0	1
Total	99	23				

Figures in brackets are numbers conceiving before marriage

(c) Courtship

In the course of the social history taken by Miss Hamilton, the mode in which the couples first met was recorded. About one third came from the same borough or immediate neighbourhood and had met at school, or in the flats or the streets of the area, or other local haunts; about a further third had met through the agency of relatives or mutual friends. In both these groups one can assume a high degree of similarity in the cultural attitudes and expectations. A further third, however, had met casually, in pubs, dance halls, while serving in the forces, or as the result of being pen pals. The chances of there being less agreement in attitudes and expectations in this latter group are clearly higher, and one might predict that this would be reflected in a poorer marital rating. The association between casual versus local encounter and the marital rating is given in *Table 13*. Although the predicted trend occurs it is far from significant. Other evidence of the possible effect of cultural discrepancy is provided by classification of

D

TABLE 13   RELATIONSHIP OF MARITAL RATING TO
HOW THE COUPLE FIRST MET

First meeting	Number	Marital rating			
		1	*2*	*3*	*4*
Casual	29	4	9	13	3
Common activity, neighbour-hood	36	6	15	13	2
Through relative or friend	25	4	12	7	2
Not known	9	1	3	4	1

the couples according to their geographical origins in *Table 14*. Again, there is a non-significant trend for couples who were both locally born and bred to be better rated. Even if this trend were significant, interpretation would be difficult in view of the probable association between migration and other social and psychiatric factors. Finally, *Table 15* records the association of discrepancies in age, social class, religion, and nationality and marital rating. None of these discrepancies shows any statistically significant associations with the marital rating, although the relationship between age discrepancy and poor adjustment is suggestive.

TABLE 14   RELATIONSHIP OF MARITAL RATING TO
GEOGRAPHICAL ORIGIN OF COUPLE

Geographical origin	Number	Marital rating			
		1	*2*	*3*	*4*
Both from the borough	45	7	21	15	2
Both from London	12	1	6	3	2
One from London, one from outside	21	4	6	10	1
Both from outside London	16	2	5	6	3
Not known	5	1	1	3	0

RELATIONSHIP BETWEEN THE 'ECONOMIC' ROLES OF THE
HUSBAND AND WIFE AND MARITAL ADJUSTMENT

One possible source of stress in marriage could be the failure of one or other partner to fulfil his or her economic tasks adequately. These

TABLE 15 RELATIONSHIP BETWEEN MARITAL RATING AND
DISCREPANCIES OF AGE, SOCIAL CLASS, PRACTISED
RELIGION, AND NATIONALITY

				Marital rating		
Disparities		*Number*	*1*	*2*	*3*	*4*
Age difference:	over 5 years	22	2	8	7	5
	under 5 years	77	13	31	30	3
Social class:	different	17	2	9	6	0
	same	82	13	30	31	8
Religion:	different	9	1	3	2	3
	same	90	14	36	35	5
Nationality:	different	16	4	3	7	2
	same	83	11	36	30	6

tasks, briefly, are for the husband to be a good provider, and for the wife to be a good housewife and manager. To investigate whether these factors were of importance, the relationship between the marital rating and the following measures was examined.

(a) The father as provider

The demand upon the father to be a good provider is a basic working-class expectation, reinforced by the memories – still vivid from the childhoods of most of our couples – of economic crisis and unemployment. In our population, however, such economic adversity had not been directly experienced in adulthood, unemployment beyond brief periods being unknown. In these conditions the ability to stick to a job provides some measure of the individual's character. Stability of employment was rated from the age of 18 or from the completion of national service on the following scale, no account being taken of changes due to the nature of the work, to promotion or to the acquisition of new skills, or of changes necessitated by rehousing:

1. *High stability:* not more than one job change in all.
2. *Medium stability:* job changes at least twice, but average interval over three years.
3. *Low stability:* job changes more often than once in three years, or more than two complete changes in occupation, unless the

past five years had been stable, in which case classify as medium.

According to this scale 74 husbands were rated High, 15 were Medium and 10 were Low. This classification bore no relationship to the marital rating. Other measures of the father as provider might be supplied by the family income and the family possessions index; both were unrelated to the marital rating.

(b) The mother as housekeeper

The efficiency of the mother as housekeeper was rated on a four-point scale by Miss Hamilton on the basis of a routine inquiry about budgeting, housekeeping methods, etc. Seventeen mothers were classified as efficient but rigid, 52 as efficient and flexible, 29 as 'happy-go-lucky' and one as disorganized. There was no significant relationship between this rating and marital adjustment. Another factor of possible importance was the employment of the mother. *Table 16* shows that mothers not at work tended to have better rated marriages, but this tendency was not significant. Were this association established, it could be interpreted either as evidence that working wives neglected their husbands or as suggesting that wives of less happy marriages were more likely to seek other rewards by going to work.

TABLE 16   RELATIONSHIP OF MARITAL RATING
TO MOTHERS' EMPLOYMENT

Mother at work	Number	Marital rating			
		1	*2*	*3*	*4*
Whole time	31	4	9	15	3
Part time	28	4	11	10	3
Not at work	40	7	19	12	2
Total	99	15	39	37	8

THE RELATIONSHIP BETWEEN THE SHARING OF TASKS
AND ACTIVITIES AND MARITAL ADJUSTMENT

There are two aspects to the division of tasks and roles: on the one hand, how the tasks are divided – who does what; and on the other hand, at least in a relatively non-structured and fluid culture, how and by whom and to whose advantage this allocation of tasks is carried out. As regards the former, information was gathered around two areas, namely responsibility for family finances and responsibility for child rearing. For each of these areas decisions were recorded as being taken either by father or by mother, or by both. As regards the latter – who allocates the tasks – no detailed investigation was made of particular issues, but a general assessment of domination and submission was carried out on each couple; this is discussed below under the heading 'Patterns of marriage'. The division of financial and child-rearing decisions in 99 couples, and the relation of this to the marital rating, is provided in *Tables 17* and *18*. Couples reporting that financial decisions were taken jointly were significantly more often well-rated (i.e. 1 or 2) on the marital rating scale ($x^2 = 8.9$, $p < 0.01$), and the same applies to joint decisions about child rearing ($x^2 = 7.5$, $p < 0.01$).

TABLE 17 RELATIONSHIP OF MARITAL RATING
TO DECISION-MAKING OVER MONEY

Decisions over money	Number	Marital rating			
		1	2	3	4
Father	22	4	7	8	3
Mother	38	3	3	18	4
Joint	39	8	19	11	1
Total	99	15	39	37	8

TABLE 18 RELATIONSHIP OF MARITAL RATING
TO DECISION-MAKING OVER CHILDREN

Decisions over children	Number	Marital rating			
		1	2	3	4
Father	12	2	3	6	1
Mother	49	5	16	21	7
Joint	38	8	20	10	0
Total	99	15	39	37	8

SOCIAL LIFE AND MARITAL ADJUSTMENT

Couples varied greatly in the degree to which they participated in social activities outside the home, either individually or as a pair. The general impression was of a population restricted in social activities and highly home-centred, where relationships of any intimacy outside the extended family were rare and where joint participation by the couple in the type of social activity so prominent in courtship – cinema-going, dancing and so on – was carried on by only a minority. The distribution of the 99 couples according to a social pattern rating and according to their joint or individual social activity was reported in Chapter 3. There was a tendency for the more integrated families (scoring 4, 5, or 6) to be better rated for marital adjustment, but this was not significant ($\chi^2 = 2 \cdot 6$, $p < 0 \cdot 2$). Individual social activity by husbands, and wives was not significantly related to the marital rating, although there was a suggestion that the wives of poorly rated marriages were more restricted. Joint activity, however, was significantly reduced in poorly rated marriages ($\chi^2 = 10 \cdot 0$, $p < 0 \cdot 01$). Although these findings relating social activity to the marital rating are only suggestive, there is certainly no evidence to suggest that the isolated couples had chosen isolation out of mutual contentment: it seems more likely that both isolation and poor marital adjustment were manifestations of a general restriction of personality.

PATTERNS OF MARRIAGE

Work on relationships in recent years has made clear the value of attempts to express them in terms of a limited number of dimensions. Most of this work is related to parent–child interactions, in which field Schaefer (1961) in particular has summarized the evidence for this approach. Others have applied a similar method in the analysis of marriage; of these Winch (1958) was of value to us in drawing up our own methods, although his theory of complementarity seems doubtfully established. It must be stated at this stage, however, that the concepts used were clarified only during the survey. This, and the absence of any objective measures – and hence a total reliance upon one observer's reports – make the analyses of marital patterns presented below unsophisticated, provisional and unvalidated. The two dimensions measured were (1) acceptance by one and dependence by the other; and (2) domination by one and submission by the other. These assessments were made upon the basis of the following definitions and criteria:

'The aim of the analysis of marital patterns is to record the current marriage relationship. While this reflects the traits of the partners, one cannot infer from looking at the marriage at one point in time how far these traits are innate to each partner and how far they are a resultant of the relationship. The description of the current relationship therefore refers to behaviour now manifest in it, or to needs expressed or inferred as existing in it currently. Needs satisfied from outside, e.g. dependence upon parents, are not scored. The two dimensions are Domination–Submission and Acceptance–Dependence; these are defined as follows:

1. Domination–submission. Domination is defined as the imposition by one partner of his or her will, needs, ideas, or interests at the expense of the other partner. Submission equals the acceptance of, or the need for, such domination. Submissive behaviour may be actively sought and/or resented at some level of consciousness at the same time. In theory, unexpressed needs for dominant or submissive behaviour may exist; in practice, each marriage may be regarded as in equilibrium or as a dominant–submissive relationship. The fact that one partner is stronger, or takes a leading role in more areas, does not imply a dominant-submissive relationship unless the strength is used to impose ascendancy and restrict the other. Marriages may therefore be in equilibrium, male-dominated, or female-dominated.

2. Acceptance–dependence. Mutual acceptance and dependence exist in every marriage. Pathological relationships occur when one partner gives tolerance, acceptance, or care for the other in a way more appropriate to the mother–child relationship, thereby imposing dependency upon the other, or when one partner demands or accepts such dependency. Theoretically, unmet needs to give acceptance can exist and are occasionally encountered; unmet dependent needs, however, are common. In practice the following groups are recognized for the purposes of classification:

(i) Mutual mature relationships.
(ii) Complementary (parent–child type) acceptance–dependence relationships.
(iii) Unmet dependent needs in one partner.
(iv) Unmet dependent needs in both partners.'

Ratings of the interview material were made according to these criteria by myself and by Miss Hamilton independently. Agreement on the domination–submission category was high, and in the cases where initial ratings were not in agreement discussion usually led to an agreed final rating without difficulty. The acceptance–dependence classification, however, proved far more difficult to apply, and differences of interpretation between the two raters occurred in too high a proportion of cases for this classification to be worth reporting in detail. In particular, it proved difficult to agree upon what constituted evidence of unsatisfied needs in one or other partner. The data showed, not surprisingly, an association between poor marital rating and the presence of unmet needs in one or both of the couple. Both mutual mature relationships, and those with complementary acceptance–dependence relationships, tended to be well rated, a finding in agreement with the clinical impression that many 'neurotic fit' marriages are reasonably successful. As regards the domination–submission category, *Table 19* demonstrates that marriages recorded as in equilibrium were most often well rated, whereas couples where the father was dominant were the worst rated. The better rating of marriages in equilibrium was significant ($\chi^2 = 21 \cdot 0$, $p < 0 \cdot 01$).

TABLE 19   RELATIONSHIP OF MARITAL RATING
TO DOMINATION

Domination/submission category	Number	Marital rating			
		1	*2*	*3*	*4*
Equilibrium	57	14	29	12	2
Father dominant	24	1	3	14	6
Mother dominant	18	0	7	11	0
Total	99	15	39	37	8

The following is an account of one of the marriages rated as a female-dominated marriage.

This couple married when the father was 30 and the mother 23. They shared household jobs and both went out to work. The main difficulties in the marriage were related by the couple to differences of temperament. Mother's main complaint was that father was insufficiently assertive or decisive: 'Where I come from,' she said, 'we expect the man to be the boss', although in fact in her own family this had not been the case. When they were first married she had looked to her husband to take the lead, but gradually she took over more and more, until she was now tending to bully and demand her own way to an ever-increasing extent. The couple discussed this at the interview. The father said, 'In the part of the world where I come from we like to be considerate; we don't like to force other people to do what we want, but my wife mistook this for weakness.' His wife denied this, but said that someone had to make up his mind, because otherwise they would still be nowhere. She complained also of his lack of ambition, whereas he complained that she seemed to have a sense of superiority, and to believe that she had been more successful than he had. She was impatient of his love of nature and music because 'it gets you nowhere'. She went on to admit that she might very well give in to their sons over things which she would refuse if the father were to ask. The father said that he knew this but had not realized that she was aware of it, to which she said, 'Well, I'm just thinking as I talk.' Their major differences concern the management of the sons, the mother deliberately undermining the father's authority. If she knows that he has said no she will almost automatically say yes, but the father, on the other hand, will never go against her; this point was in fact underlined by one of the sons who was present for part of the interview. When differences of opinion arise, father likes to set out all the detailed reasons, but finally, in the face of her 'hysterics', he invariably gives in. On one occasion he had slapped her face when she was creating a scene, but he felt bad about it afterwards, and quite soon apologized. She is prone to sulk, in which case he invariably tries to win her round. Father was the more obviously affectionate of the two and was more prepared to accept and tolerate her than she was him. Nevertheless, there did seem to be some underlying mutual friendliness between them, at least when they were not arguing.

DURATION OF MARRIAGE

As this study was made at one point in time, no very accurate impression can be given of the development of marital relationships through time. However, it was possible to compare marriages of greater duration with those of lesser duration; this is done in *Table 20*, where the population is divided into those married more or less than twelve years. It should be noted that very few couples had been married less than six years. It is seen from this table that marriages of greater duration were worse rated. This sad association is statistically significant ($\chi^2 = 5\cdot0$, $p < 0\cdot05$).

TABLE 20 RELATIONSHIP OF MARITAL RATING
TO DURATION OF MARRIAGE

		Marital rating			
Duration of marriage	Number	1	2	3	4
Less than 12 years	55	9	27	15	4
More than 12 years	44	6	12	22	4
Total	99	15	39	37	8

BROKEN OR NON-ESTABLISHED MARRIAGES

In the account so far, no mention has been made of those families in which there was only one parent at the time of the survey, and no account has been given of the previous marital histories of the present parents. As failure to achieve or sustain a marriage, and the consequent disruption of family life, is an event of major significance for the children, some details will now be provided, first, of the single-parent families, secondly, of those in second marriages, and, thirdly, of developments in the period since the survey up to the time of writing.

Single-parent families

At the time of the survey, eleven of the 112 families were headed by the mother alone and two by the father alone. The economic problems of these families were indicated in Chapter 2. In four of these cases the other parent had died – three fathers and one mother; of these, two of the fathers had not been legally married to the mothers, having had previous undissolved marriages, and being considerably older than the mothers. Two other families were headed by women who had never cohabited with the fathers: in one, conception occurred during an engagement which was broken off by the father; in the other the woman had had a long-term irregular liaison with a married man by whom she had three children, having left her own husband (with one child) some years before. Of the remaining seven families the parents had separated in three (in one case the mother had already had a child before the marriage), and were divorced in

58

four. Among the families with two parents at the time of the survey there were two where both parents had had previous marriages; in one further couple the husband had lost his first wife through death, and had remarried, the child of the first marriage being incorporated in the second family. In another couple the eldest child was an illegitimate child of the mother by another man, born two years before the marriage. Between the survey interviews and the time of writing, an average interval of two years, two more families had lost one parent by death – one father and one mother – but two parents who had been on their own had remarried. Four further couples had separated or divorced in this period; in one of these cases the couple were not legally married but had cohabited for fourteen years. The marital ratings accorded to the four couples who had separated since the survey were 4, 4, 3, and 2; the last couple were a neurotic, immature pair, who had appeared at the time of the interview to have a reasonably stable, 'neurotic fit' relationship, but the mother's psychiatric state had worsened considerably in the ensuing two years.

Some form of marital disruption was therefore seen to be very common in our survey population. At the time of writing, only 87 of the 112 families were headed by two parents, legally married, with no previous marriage or pregnancy. Our sample of primary school children, by selection, excluded cases of total family breakdown where the children were in care. As further disruptions may be confidently predicted it seems likely that about one quarter of the children will have been deprived for part of their childhood of the stable and continuous care of both parents. To assess the effect of this, however, is by no means easy, the age of the child at the time of disruption being an important variable and the antecedents of the disruption being varied and often themselves traumatic.

From the point of view of social policy, disruption due to death cannot be avoided, but separation and divorce are less inevitable. In case anybody were to conclude that a reduction in their frequency – say by making divorce more difficult – might be beneficial, some details of those separated and divorced are provided.

In the four couples divorced before the time of the survey, the divorced partner had exhibited abnormal behaviour in three: sexual deviation in one father, psychopathic and at times sadistic behaviour in another, sexual interference with his daughters and rape of his wife in the third; in the fourth case the wife had a deeply neurotic personality. Of the three cases of separation, the parents now with the children were all unstable, one mother having had a severe chronic anxiety state for which several periods of hospitalization had been required. Of the four couples separating since the survey, one pair were immature and neurotic (mentioned above), in one non-legal union the father was a problem drinker and frequently physically violent, and in the remaining two there were sadomasochistic-type relationships with bullying, infidelity, and violence on the husbands' part and neurotic symptoms in the wives. Clearly, any attempt to blame the fact of divorce or separation for any disturbance in the children of these couples would be unrealistic: the divorce or separation in every case was a manifestation of long-standing disturbance of relationships and of personalities.

THE MARRIAGE RELATIONSHIP AND NEUROSIS

Many of the factors already discussed in relation to marital adjustment are also known to bear a relationship to the childhood experience of the individual, which in turn is related to neuroticism. It is difficult, therefore, to extract from all these factors the relative importance of the marriage itself compared with these associated influences. However, certain associations between marriage and neurosis are of particular interest, and in this section an attempt will be made to answer three questions, namely how far husbands and wives resemble each other in respect of neuroticism, how far marital adjustment and neuroticism are related, and how far is marital failure associated with neuroticism. The relevant figures are summarized in *Tables 21* and *22*.

Neurosis in husbands and wives

There was a significant tendency for husbands and wives to resemble each other in respect of neuroticism (using the 'minimal neurosis' criterion, $\chi^2 = 8 \cdot 1$, $p < 0 \cdot 01$). This resemblance could represent either assortative mating or the result of interaction. In couples already married for several years we have no direct evidence about personality or neuroticism prior to marriage. There was, however, no evidence for any correlation between the recollected childhoods of husbands and their wives, which is perhaps evidence against selection. This point is discussed further in the next section.

TABLE 21 MINIMAL NEUROSIS IN MOTHERS RELATED TO OWN
CHILDHOOD, HUSBAND'S CHILDHOOD, AND MARITAL RATING

Childhood experience			Husband's childhood			Marital rating		
	No.	Minimal neurosis		No.	Minimal neurosis	Rating	No.	Minimal neurosis
Secure	42	26 (62%)	Secure	28	16 (57%)	1 or 2	20	9 (45%)
						3 or 4	8	7 (88%)
			Adverse	14	10 (71%)	1 or 2	7	4 (57%)
						3 or 4	7	6 (86%)
Adverse	57	50 (88%)	Secure	34	31 (91%)	1 or 2	16	14 (88%)
						3 or 4	18	17 (94%)
			Adverse	23	19 (83%)	1 or 2	11	7 (64%)
						3 or 4	12	12 (100%)

TABLE 22 MINIMAL NEUROSIS IN FATHERS RELATED TO OWN
CHILDHOOD, WIFE'S CHILDHOOD, AND MARITAL RATING

Childhood experience			Wife's childhood			Marital rating		
	No.	Minimal neurosis		No.	Minimal neurosis	Rating	No.	Minimal neurosis
Secure	62	27 (43%)	Secure	28	10 (36%)	1 or 2	20	6 (30%)
						3 or 4	8	4 (50%)
			Adverse	34	17 (50%)	1 or 2	16	9 (56%)
						3 or 4	18	8 (44%)
Adverse	37	23 (62%)	Secure	14	7 (50%)	1 or 2	7	4 (57%)
						3 or 4	7	13 (43%)
			Adverse	23	16 (70%)	1 or 2	11	5 (45%)
						3 or 4	12	11 (92%)

Marital adjustment and neurosis

An association between neurosis and poor marital adjustment was
shown for both sexes but reached significance only in the case of the
wives, where a rating of 3 or 4 on the marital adjustment scale was
significantly associated with minimal neurosis ($\chi^2 = 11 \cdot 0$, $p < 0 \cdot 01$).
This association might be explained in terms of personality structure
(neurotic people making immature relationships), or in terms of re-
action to current stress (a disturbed relationship provoking neurotic

symptoms). It is likely that both processes occur. In *Tables 21* and *22*, the population is classified according to minimal neurosis, marital adjustment, and the childhood experience of both the individual and the spouse. These tables suggest that a poor marital rating may be related to minimal neurosis independently of the effects of childhood experience, at least in the case of women; the tables also show that adverse childhood experience of one spouse was related to minimal neurosis in the other. Although this finding was not significant, it suggests that at least some of the husband–wife resemblance in respect of neurosis may be the effect of interaction rather than of selection. This point was discussed in our paper (Pond *et al.*, 1963). Evidence for an effect of interaction was found by Kreitman (1964) in a hospital-based study.

Marital failure and neurosis

The relationship between a poor marital rating and neurosis, already described, is repeated in respect of marital failure. Marital failure for this purpose is taken to include a history of separation or divorce, including those occurring since the survey, or of previous marriage or conception, or the non-establishment of a legal union. Thirteen women and five men are in this category. From *Table 23* it is seen that all these individuals met the criteria for minimal neurosis.

TABLE 23   MARITAL FAILURE AND NEUROSIS

Parent		Number	Minimal neurosis	No. with C.M.I. 31+	C.M.I. not completed
Women:	Marital failure	13	13	7	2
	No marital failure	97	69	20	2
Men:	Marital failure	5	5	2	2
	No marital failure	96	46	12	1

SUMMARY

In forming generalizations from a population one is forced to fit cases into categories, and to reduce complex and uncertain phenomena to rating and scores. This process, however unsatisfactory, has demonstrated that in this population marriages which were judged satisfactory were characterized by a better rating for communication, better sexual adjustment, by more sharing of decisions, more joint social activity, and by fewer domination–submission conflicts. Couples who had both experienced secure childhoods tended to be better married, but youth at marriage and premarital conception were not related to marital adjustment. Husbands and wives tended to be similar in respect of neuroticism, and poor marital adjustment was associated with neurosis (significant only for women). Individuals who had failed in their marriages all met the criteria of minimal neurosis.

It is obvious that the marriage relationship provides both a source and an indicator of an individual's maturity and stability. More detailed investigations into the relationship between psychiatric illness and marital behaviour would clearly be desirable. Meanwhile, this is obviously an aspect of family life which is of direct relevance to any study of the child's environment.

CHAPTER 6

Child-rearing Practices and their
Relation to other Parental Attributes

The thoughtlessness, carelessness, and cocksureness with
which children are brought up is frightful to see: and yet
everyone is essentially what they are to be when they are ten
years old; and yet one would find that almost everyone bears
with them a defect from their childhood, which they do not
overcome even in their seventieth year; together with the fact
that all unhappy individualities are related to a false impression received in childhood.

Oh, piteous satire upon mankind; that providence should
have endowed almost every child so richly because it knew in
advance what was to befall it: to be brought up by 'parents',
i.e. to be made a mess of in every possible way.

The journals of Kierkegaard (translated by A. Dru)

No mother is so wicked but desires to have good children.

Italian proverb

The social and marital state of the population has been described in
the preceding chapters, and the incidence and some associations of
neurosis in the parents have been discussed. While all these factors
are obviously of relevance in the child's development, the direct study
of the child-rearing attitudes and practices of the parents remains to
be reported. There is a huge literature and output of research on the
relationship of parental behaviour to symptoms of emotional disturbance in the child. The problems and limitations of this work
have been ably summarized by Spiegel and Bell (1959) who, after
reviewing the achievements and deficiencies of much of the work in
this field, write as follows:

'... the weight of the evidence, in spite of the lack of control groups,
points to *some* relationship between the unconscious motivation
and overt behaviour of the parents and the emotional difficulties
of the child. One may well ask what needs to be done in order to

clear up the vagueness and confusion about the precise nature of this relationship which presently characterizes the literature. At the very least, it would seem apparent that the confusion will persist as long as investigators attend only to partial relationships within the family.'

In the present chapter, the methods used to rate parental attitudes and behaviour are reported, and the relation between child-rearing practices and some other parental attributes is examined. The relationship of these measures of parental behaviour to psychological disturbance in the child is discussed in Chapter 8.

Two main methods were used to measure child-rearing practices: rating of interview material, and parent-attitude questionnaires.

INTERVIEW ASSESSMENT OF PARENTAL ATTITUDES

The fact that one and the same observer was collecting data both on psychological disturbance in the child and on the child-rearing practices of the parents meant that the possibility of bias, based upon assumed interrelations, was ever present. In an effort to guard against this, ratings of parental behaviour were based upon the parents' accounts of their beliefs and behaviour, and not upon inferences about their attitudes. If it seemed at interview that 'acceptable' attitudes were being expressed, further questioning would sometimes produce confirmatory evidence of suspected underlying attitudes. But such questioning was not always considered justifiable in the context of a research interview, and hence in some cases attitudes and behaviour may have been suspected but, as descriptions were not elicited, these attitudes were not rated.

The accounts of this part of the interview were rated against a number of scales of our own construction. These scales were unrealistically elaborate, and the scoring methods used are open to criticism. The main use made of them is to provide: (1) a score of *acceptance* (classified into adequate and low) derived from five separate scales; (2) a classification on the basis of one scale of *parental discipline* into strict, intermediate and lax; (3) a classification on the basis of one scale of *parental consistency*. Independent rating (by myself) of the interview material on these scales showed very good agreement with Miss Hamilton's ratings. The classification derived, despite the methodological weaknesses, is, I believe, reasonably valid. Details of the scales, the scoring methods and score distributions are provided in the appendix to this chapter.

One further rating was made by Miss Hamilton: an assessment of whether the parents displayed neurotic involvement with their children, such as projection, displacement, or over-identification. This rating was clearly open to the danger of bias due to knowledge of the child, but was always backed up with supporting evidence.

The interrelationships of parent-attitude ratings

These are summarized in *Tables 24* and *25*. Too few parents were rated as lax disciplinarians to draw conclusions about the relationship of this to other attitudes. Strict disciplinarians, however, were significantly more likely to be rated low for acceptance (mothers $\chi^2 = 25$, fathers $\chi^2 = 14$, $p < 0.01$). Parents judged to show neurotic involvement with their children were liable to be rated low for acceptance (fathers $\chi^2 = 4.4$, $p < 0.05$, mothers $\chi^2 = 3.3$, $p < 0.01$) and they were also likely to be rated as strict disciplinarians (fathers $\chi^2 = 3.5$, $p < 0.1$, mothers $\chi^2 = 24$, $p < 0.01$). Low acceptance and low consis-

TABLE 24 ACCEPTANCE AND DOMINATION CLASSIFICATION OF 110 MOTHERS RELATED TO RATINGS FOR CONSISTENCY AND FOR NEUROTIC INVOLVEMENT WITH THE CHILD

| Acceptance | Domination | No. | Consistency rating | | | | | Neurotic involvement with child | |
			1 (High)	2	3	4	5 (Low)	Yes (+ or ++)	No
Adequate	High	10	1	0	8	0	1	8	2
	Intermediate	35	13	1	21	0	0	10	25
	Low	12	1	0	11	0	0	7	5
	Combined	57	15	1	40	0	1	25	32
Low	High	25	0	5	14	4	2	22	3
	Intermediate	16	5	0	10	1	0	7	9
	Low	12	0	0	8	3	1	7	5
	Combined	53	5	5	32	8	3	36	17
Total	Combined	110	20	6	72	8	4	61	49

tency were related in mothers ($\chi^2 = 8\cdot5, p < 0\cdot01$). These interrelationships reflect, of course, the relation between the judgements of a single observer, and the different ratings cannot be regarded as independent variables.

TABLE 25 ACCEPTANCE AND DOMINATION CLASSIFICATION OF 100 FATHERS RELATED TO RATINGS FOR CONSISTENCY AND FOR NEUROTIC INVOLVEMENT WITH THE CHILD

			Consistency rating					Neurotic involvement with child	
			1	*2*	*3*	*4*	*5*	*Yes*	*No*
Acceptance	*Domination*	*No.*	*(High)*				*(Low)*	*(+ or ++)*	
Adequate	High	4	2	2	0	0	0	4	0
	Intermediate	49	40	4	5	0	0	5	44
	Low	6	2	0	4	0	0	4	2
	Combined	59	44	6	9	0	0	13	46
Low	High	21	0	10	6	4	1	10	11
	Intermediate	17	6	2	8	1	0	7	10
	Low	3	0	0	0	0	3	1	2
	Combined	41	6	12	14	5	4	18	23
Total	Combined	100	50	18	23	5	4	31	69

The following two case records, selected at random, illustrate the type of material upon which these ratings were based.

1. The Leslie family
This family consisted of mother and father; Elizabeth, aged 15; and John, the survey child, aged eight.

Mother: General attitude. She said she particularly liked John's good manners and gratitude, also his attentive concern for her. His tempers made her angry partly because she felt helpless in the face of them and partly they embarrassed her – 'he shows you up'. She described him as 'terribly affectionate' and clearly revelled in this. From seeing them together it seems that she probably gets some erotic satisfaction. With Elizabeth she had 'rigid rules' and Elizabeth always obeyed without question; John, however, would argue his point and mother very often gave in. She also allowed him to go too far, varying with her mood as to how far she would let him go, and then might suddenly lose her temper, shouting and hitting him around the legs. Sometimes she would threaten 'wait for your father'. She was quite critical, would tell John off if he did not come up to scratch, and she would 'go off' at Elizabeth, for instance when she did not do her room out properly. She wondered if perhaps she expected too much of the children for their ages. At John's age, Elizabeth was expected to do many household chores but nothing was demanded of John except for occasional errands – 'he seems such a baby'. For this reason, too, she was over-protective, doing more for him than he needed and worrying if he was out of her sight. The fact that she still took him to school, however, seemed reasonable in view of the distance he had to go. She spent a great deal of time with him every evening drawing, playing with him, doing quizzes, etc. She said she really enjoyed this but also commented 'it passes the time, particularly on father's late turns'.

Father: General attitude. He said he was satisfied with John the way he was except that he was too babyish. He held that showing affection made children babyish and for that reason he had never done so with either of his children. Elizabeth in fact had never asked for it, but John had done, and father had always pushed him off. However, it seems that in other ways John has managed to draw father out. Mother said he used to hide himself consistently behind a book but now would sometimes take notice of John and help him make models or other things. This was a fairly recent development and the time he actually gave to him was really very little and irregular, strictly depending on his mood. With Elizabeth he would sometimes not speak for days on end but did not do this with John, as John took no notice and continued to try and draw father out. If father thought he had been unjust he could apologize even to Elizabeth, though he admitted that this was sometimes very hard. When asked his opinion of praising children he said he was all for it – he thought it encouraged them and he was carrying on in this vein when mother interrupted him saying 'yes, but you never think of doing it, do you', at which he rather ruefully agreed that perhaps he didn't. He was very firm and John knew it was no good insisting – 'he won't try to push to the limit' but did what he was told the first time. Very occasionally father might make exceptions. He very rarely hit, his main punishment being to put to bed. The last time he had done this it was on account of temper and swearing, some months ago. He didn't worry much over John and thought that he should learn to find his own way about; if mother was doubtful, his attitude was 'let him go'.

These parents never actually went against each other, but what usually happened was that John would ask mother first; she would not say yes outright, but in fact would have every intention of persuading father to give the final word yes. If father had already said no she was likely to go in with John and say, 'Did you say he couldn't do so and so?' and would then put forward good reasons why it should be allowed. Father would often stick to his no at first but would often be persuaded by mother's arguments. It seemed that there was certainly no doubt in John's mind that mother was his ally. Sometimes father would tell John to get off his mother's lap, and there had been quite serious rows between them over mother's alleged babying of the boy.

Classification by the scales: It was considered that the mother showed marked neurotic involvement with the boy and that the father did not. Mother's parent attitude classification was: acceptance – adequate; discipline – strict; consistency – variable.

Father's classification was: acceptance – low; discipline – strict; consistency – unpredictable.

2. The Armstrong family

This family consists of father; mother; and Shirley, aged 10½ at the time of the survey interview.

Mother: General Attitude. Mother had decisive ideas about the upbringing of children, but several times said in parenthesis 'perhaps I'm hard, but that's the way I think', or 'you'll think I'm unsympathetic'. She had very high standards, expected certain duties of Shirley about the house, and did not hesitate to criticize if they did not come up to her standard – 'I'm not one for handing out praise, I'm afraid.' She was not naturally demonstrative and was sometimes irritated when Shirley chose the wrong moment to show her affection. At other times she could respond to the child's overtures. One thing she would not tolerate was rudeness or cheek in any form, and she would not hesitate to smack or send Shirley to her bedroom for this. She also tended to shout rather and admitted that she probably could be said to nag. She never bribed or rewarded and refused to increase pocket money or school money, although she knew that the majority of children had more than Shirley: 'you'll think I'm hard, but it was the way I was brought up.' Although she knew she was erratic and had irritable moods she did not think that her handling of Shirley varied a great deal: certain things were allowed or not allowed, and what varied was the vehemence with which her word was enforced. The parents tried not to interfere with each other's authority, although each might try to temper the other's discipline, occasionally in front of the child but more often afterwards. Mother was the stricter of the two and did most checking, but on the other hand she was the more flexible. She liked Shirley to be capable, allowed her to experiment, and let her come and go without worrying unduly. She spent quite a bit of time with her, playing games in the evenings, going swimming with her, etc.

Father: General attitude. He had fewer rules than mother but was firm and rather rigid about these. He very rarely hit Shirley, but he might raise his voice to her and Shirley was then much more likely to cry than she was with all mother's nagging. He was more demonstrative than mother and more ready to hand out praise and to show appreciation. He showed as much interest in her doings as did the mother and spent time most evenings talking to her or playing games. He would not tolerate cheek in any form. Although he allowed Shirley to come and go freely he probably worried a bit more about her than mother.

Classification by the scales: It was felt on balance that there was evidence of neurotic involvement in the mother's attitudes. She had given other evidence of difficulty in accepting feminine roles, a difficulty probably stemming from her own childhood experience of divorced parents and an alcoholic mother, and it was felt that some of her strict control of Shirley therefore represented projection. Mother's classification on the attitude scales was: acceptance – low;

discipline – intermediate; consistency – consistent and flexible.

Father's was: acceptance – adequate; discipline – intermediate; consistency – consistent and rigid.

QUESTIONNAIRE ASSESSMENT OF PARENTAL ATTITUDES

Some time after the survey interviews, questionnaires were sent out to all the parents. The mothers' questionnaire, designed to measure both acceptance and domination, was designed by Dr Oppenheim of the London School of Economics, and had already been administered by him to a large population. The scores for domination and acceptance used in our survey were derived from three sub-scales of this inventory (*democracy, autocracy, acceptance*) on the basis of Dr Oppenheim's analysis of his initial pilot administration of the inventory, which showed that these sub-scales correlated closely with the scores for domination and acceptance derived from the whole instrument. Acceptance was classified as low (scores 19 or less on the acceptance scale) or adequate. Domination was classified as high (32 or more), intermediate, or low (22 or less) according to a score derived from the autocracy and democracy scores (the score being derived as the autocracy score plus 30 minus the democracy score). The score distributions are given in the appendix to this chapter.

The fathers' questionnaire, designed by Dr Gibson of the Camberwell Family Study, measured domination only. This test was still undergoing development at the time of administration, the fathers in our population in fact providing part of the pilot population, and two versions of the instrument being used. Because of this, details of the scoring methods and cut-off points are not reproduced here. The scores were used, as in the case of the mothers, to give a classification of domination as high, intermediate, or low.

THE RELATIONSHIP OF THE TWO ASSESSMENTS
OF PARENTAL ATTITUDES

Inspection of the acceptance classification according to the interview and inventory showed no apparent relation between the two. Correlation coefficients for these two scores were calculated for the population subdivided according to the consistency rating and according to the score on the C.M.I., to see if either of these factors might have introduced distortion in either instrument and hence have decreased agreement. However, the correlation coefficients obtained did not differ significantly with these factors, and the highest correlation obtained for any group was 0·14. The domination classifications by interview and inventory, given in *Table 26*, were similarly virtually unrelated in the case of mothers; in the case of fathers there is some slight non-significant trend towards agreement.

TABLE 26   A COMPARISON OF THE CLASSIFICATION OF 110 MOTHERS AND 100 FATHERS BY THE INTERVIEW AND INVENTORY RATINGS FOR DOMINATION

Domination by interview	Domination by inventory							
	Mothers				Fathers			
	High	Inter-mediate	Low	Not done	High	Inter-mediate	Low	Not done
High	10	21	2	2	8	10	1	6
Intermediate	9	27	9	6	14	30	9	13
Low	6	13	0	5	0	3	3	3

Although some discrepancy between an interview rating of behaviour and an inventory rating of attitudes would be predicted, the total failure to correlate is surprising. Crandall and Preston (1955), for example, showed fair agreement between mothers' self ratings for affection and ratings applied by psychologists. The inventories used in our study had not been validated against clinical ratings or against other measures such as the child's perception of his parents. The variations by social class reported by Pitfield and Oppenheim (1964) on their instrument may have reflected differences in social desirability sets rather than differences in behaviour.

In the remaining part of this chapter, both interview and inventory measures will be related to some other parental attributes. Meanwhile, the following six excerpts are taken from the records of mothers who scored at opposite extremes of the range for acceptance by interview and inventory. They would seem to offer good evidence for the interview rating, and my own inclination is to accept these as probably more valid.

*I: Mothers scoring high for acceptance by inventory
and low by interview*

1. Mrs A said at first, 'I wouldn't have her different but I can't stand cheek'. Her attitude varied in fact with her mood, but whatever her mood dictated she would not retract subsequently. She was observed at the interview to be anxious for the child to do her credit, and tended to be naggingly critical to that end. She used to throw the child's paintings away as 'rubbish', and was quite undemonstrative towards the child, while demanding comfort and support from her.

2. Mrs B seemed aloof at interview, her comments on the child being largely critical, e.g. that he was spoilt by his father, was stubborn, was lazy, had a nasty temper. She was able to praise for jobs well done but was frequently discouraging because of his slowness. She shouted at him a great deal, quite often hit him, and worried very little about him when he was out.

3. Mrs C was rather placating, using many bribes and rewards. She was not demonstrative to the child and gave very little time to her – 'I seem to be too busy.' She restricted the child in doing jobs because she didn't do them well. While fussing about the child, she did not in fact meet her demands for attention.

*II: Mothers rated high for acceptance on interview
but low on inventory*

1. Mrs D described herself as 'not naturally demonstrative'. She did, however, show warmth in her general attitude. She seemed to handle the youngest child in a tender, motherly way. She tried to get to know the children in their own different ways, was interested in showing them how to do things, and when they were successful was ready to praise them.

2. Mrs E was very accepting and understanding in speaking of and dealing with the children. She seemed warmly affectionate by nature, ready to praise without expecting too high a standard, tending to be somewhat over-protective. She spent much time playing with them and helping with their games.

3. Mrs F spoke in an accepting way, showing good understanding of the differences between her children. She was prepared to be equally demonstrative to all and protected the children from their father's teasing. She would soon praise their efforts, having shown them how to do things, and was able to let them try without

interference. She spent a great deal of time both in playing with them and in taking them out on excursions, and really seemed to enjoy her children.

THE RELATIONSHIP OF PARENTAL ATTITUDES AND BEHAVIOUR TO OTHER PARENTAL ATTRIBUTES

Bearing in mind the comments of Spiegel and Bell referred to at the beginning of this chapter, it seemed of interest to see whether our ratings of parental attitudes and behaviour showed any significant relationship with other characteristics of the parents. Three parental characteristics were selected for study, namely neuroticism as measured by the C.M.I., poor marital adjustment, and a history of adverse childhood experience (rated as described in Chapter 3). It was considered that these three factors might provide some reflection of possible immaturity or of psychological defences, which in turn might influence child-rearing practices. More specifically it was predicted that neurotic, poorly married individuals with adverse childhood experience would tend as parents to show low acceptance and extremes, either high or low, of domination.

TABLE 27 ACCEPTANCE AND DOMINATION CLASSIFICATION OF 110 MOTHERS RELATED TO CHILDHOOD EXPERIENCE, MARITAL RATING, AND C.M.I. SCORE

Accep-tance	Domination	No.	Childhood experience		Marital rating				C.M.I. score		
			Ad-verse	Se-cure	1 or 2	3	4	5	0–30	31+	Not done
Adequate	High	10	7	3	7	3	0	0	4	5	1
	Inter-mediate	35	18	17	21	11	0	3	24	11	0
	Low	12	10	2	3	8	1	0	5	6	1
	Combined	57	35	22	31	22	1	3	33	22	2
Low	High	25	16	9	12	4	5	4	15	8	2
	Inter-mediate	16	9	7	8	5	1	2	13	3	0
	Low	12	5	7	3	6	1	2	7	5	0
	Combined	53	30	23	23	15	7	8	35	16	2
Total	Combined	110	65	45	54	37	8	11	68	38	4

Some of these predictions were borne out in the case of the interview ratings. The findings are summarized in *Tables 27* and *28*.

TABLE 28 ACCEPTANCE AND DOMINATION CLASSIFICATION OF 100 FATHERS RELATED TO CHILDHOOD EXPERIENCE, MARITAL RATING, AND C.M.I. SCORE

Accep-tance	Domination	No.	Childhood experience		Marital rating				C.M.I. score		
			Ad-verse	Se-cure	1 or 2	3	4	5	0–30	31+	Not done
Adequate	High	4	1	3	3	0	0	1	3	1	0
	Inter-mediate	49	12	37	30	17	2	0	44	4	1
	Low	6	1	5	3	3	0	0	6	0	0
	Combined	59	14	45	36	20	2	1	52	5	1
Low	High	21	12	9	10	8	2	1	16	3	2
	Inter-mediate	17	10	7	7	8	2	0	14	3	0
	Low	3	2	1	0	1	2	0	0	3	0
	Combined	41	24	17	17	17	6	1	30	9	2
Total	Combined	100	38	62	53	37	8	2	82	14	3

Low acceptance was significantly associated with adverse childhood experience in fathers ($\chi^2 = 11$, $p < 0.01$) but not in mothers. A marital rating of 4 or 5 was associated with low acceptance in both parents (fathers $\chi^2 = 3.6$, $p < 0.1$, mothers $\chi^2 = 7.3$, $p < 0.01$). The C.M.I. score, however, showed no association with the acceptance rating. None of these three factors showed any relationship with the rating for domination.

There was only one association of these parental characteristics with the inventory classification for acceptance and domination. This was between adverse childhood and high domination in fathers, and this association was significant at the 10 per cent level only.

THE RELATIONSHIP BETWEEN PARENTAL ATTITUDES
AND BEHAVIOUR OF HUSBANDS AND WIVES

There was no significant tendency for husbands to resemble their wives in respect of either domination or acceptance ratings by inventory or interview assessments.

DISCUSSION

It is obvious in retrospect that the methodological problems encountered in rating behaviour could have been tackled in many better ways, including, for example, the use of independent interviewing for the recording of data on the child's psychological state and the parents' attitudes (this would have increased the expense considerably), and the recording of the child's perception of the parent rather than, or in addition to, the direct recording of parental attitudes (Andry, 1960; Kagan, 1956; Bene and Anthony, 1957; Ausubel *et al.*, 1954). Beyond this one should perhaps consider how far measures of domination and acceptance are adequate and meaningful, or whether the balance between them may not matter more than the level of either, or whether other dimensions such as the degree of confidence shown by the parents may not be of more significance (see Gildea *et al.*, 1961), or whether other processes, such as identification and imitation, or the transmission of patterns of interaction (Henry, 1951), may not be areas equally deserving study and measurement.

Granted the limitations, if our interview classification is accepted as to some degree valid, the relation of adverse child-rearing attitudes to adverse childhood or marital experience is suggestive, serving to emphasize that the origins of a child's psychological state are unlikely to be found by studying only one parent or only one aspect of one parent. We can claim to have provided some epidemiological support for the clinical conviction that a parent's impact upon a child is likely to be inextricably linked with his or her history, personality, and marriage relationship.

APPENDIX TO CHAPTER 6
RATING METHODS

A. Rating scales of acceptance

The following five scales relating to acceptance were used, in the belief that the form of acceptance might vary between fathers and mothers and between different individuals. Scores on these scales were allotted around an 'ideal' level of 5, higher scores indicating smothering or over-protectiveness, lower scores a degree of rejection. (This arbitrary weighting is open to criticism.)

1. Acceptance–rejection

5: Accepting and insightful.

4: Accepts child much as he is, but little insight or imaginative understanding.

3: Acceptance conditional on child's behaviour or degree of tolerance and understanding of child.

2: Intolerant and insensitive to needs.

1: Harshly rejecting, uncaring.

2. Demonstrative affection

7: Very demonstrative. Affection lavished. Does not leave child alone.

5: Warmly responsive to child's need for affection.

3: Demonstrative at times, dependent on mood, circumstances, etc.

2: Seldom demonstrates affection.

1: Cold, withdrawn.

3. Practical evidence of affection

7: Encroachment of child's needs and interests to exclusion of those of parents. Some excess of expenditure to meet child's demands or supposed needs. Doting.

5: Enjoys child's company and enters co-operatively into daily interests and activities, but balance kept between child and adult needs. Wise, considered expenditure on child's behalf.

   3: Occasionally/irregularly spares time to be with child, make/ mend toys, etc. or deliberately sets time aside out of sense of duty. Some lack of generosity in providing for child's needs.

   2: Indulgent provision of material things in lieu of personal interest and time.

   1: Little or no thought, time, or money devoted to child and/or his interest.

4. *Esteem-building*

   7: Praises indiscriminately, child can do no wrong.

   5: Praises for achievement, encourages self-reliance and independence. Tries to mitigate inadequacies and failures.

   3: Praises or rewards for good behaviour, but blames and criticizes inadequacies and errors, i.e. for failing to reach parental standards. 'Emotional blackmail'.

   2: Disparages or belittles child's attempts. Takes tasks out of his hands in well-meant attempt to help, or impatient at incompetence. Well-meant teasing which child understands as ridicule.

   1: Consistently disparages and ridicules. Prefers child to be dependent and undermines confidence to this end.

5. *Over-protection/Neglect*

   7: Grossly over-protective, smothering.

   6: Over-protective, inadequate freedom for child to experiment.

   5: Average. Normal concern.

   3: Somewhat neglectful.

   1: Gross neglect (child's need for attention and encouragement not met).

The score on Scale 1 correlated with the sum scores from Scales 2–5 in a sample of 30 mothers and 28 fathers at the level $r = 0.70$. Score distribution of the population on the acceptance score derived from these scales is given in *Table I* of this appendix.

TABLE I DISTRIBUTION OF ACCEPTANCE SCORES, ASSESSED BY
INTERVIEW OF 110 MOTHERS AND 100 FATHERS

Acceptance classification	*Low*			*Adequate*			
Acceptance score	15 or less	16–17	18–19	20–21	22–23	24–25	26 or more
Mothers' score distribution	9	22	22	13	20	19	5
Fathers' score distribution	17	9	15	14	20	21	4

A score of 0–19 was classified as low, one of 20 or more as adequate. As exception may well be taken to this scoring method an alternative classification was carried out on the following basis. Any individual who was not rated below the third scale position on any of the five scales, and who was rated on the first or second position on at least two scales, was classified as adequate, and the remainder were classified as low. *Table II* compares the classification so obtained with that derived from the sum scores and shows a reasonably high degree of agreement.

TABLE II COMPARISON OF ACCEPTANCE
CLASSIFICATION DERIVED FROM TWO DIFFERENT
METHODS (FATHERS AND MOTHERS COMBINED)

Classification by scale positions	*Classification by summed scores*	
	Adequate	*Low*
Adequate	102	7
Low	14	87

B. Rating of parental discipline

The *parental discipline* scale, and the distribution of parents upon it, is as follows:

Score	Fathers	Mothers	
7	0	0	Child's movements are dictated by the parents with virtually no exercise of choice possible.

Score	Fathers	Mothers	
6	25	35	Child's area of choice limited in a way inappropriate to its maturity; limits arbitrarily defined by the parents' conscious or unconscious needs rather than by the child's needs or by the reality of the situation.
4	66	51	Child given freedom within the limits of its maturity; explanations within limits of its comprehension; firm limits being set upon permitted behaviour.
2	7	24	Child given more freedom of choice than is appropriate for age and circumstances, the bounds of permitted behaviour being poorly defined.
1	2	0	No formal disciplinary framework provided. Licence or complete lack of interest from parents – virtually abandoned all attempt to control the child.

It is seen that this was a poorly designed scale, giving virtually a three-point assessment. Points 1 and 2 were classified as strict, 3 as intermediate, 4 and 5 as lax.

C. A rating of consistency

The distribution of scores on this scale are given in *Tables 24* and *25* (pp. 66, 67). The scale items read as follows:

5: Very consistent but flexible. Child knows where he is but can expect exceptions.

4: Very consistent but rigid; won't go back on word regardless of circumstances.

3: Consistency varies according to parent's mood, circumstances, or child's insistence, but child may be able to predict.

2: Generally unpredictable. May be constant in one or two respects.

1: Totally unpredictable. Alternations of extremes – harshness/indulgence, uncontrolled fury/guilt reactions.

D. *Inventory ratings of mothers' attitudes*
The score distributions are given in *Tables III* and *IV* of this appendix.

TABLE III   ACCEPTANCE SCORE DISTRIBUTION OF 97 MOTHERS
ON THE INVENTORY

Acceptance classification	*Low*				*Adequate*				
Acceptance score	16 or less	17	18	19	20	21	22	23	24 or more
Number of mothers	11	9	9	8	20	10	9	16	5

TABLE IV   DOMINATION SCORE DISTRIBUTION OF 97 MOTHERS
ON THE INVENTORY

Domination classification	*Low*				*Intermediate*									*High*		
Domination score[1]	19 or less	20	21	22	23	24	25	26	27	28	29	30	31	32	33	34 or more
Number of mothers	3	1	0	6	6	4	6	9	10	3	11	6	7	9	6	10

[1]Based on two sub-scales of Dr Oppenheim's inventory: the c (democracy) and b (autocracy) scale. Score $= 30—c+b$.

CHAPTER 7

Psychological Disturbance in the Children

> They are bound to have the defects of their qualities.
>
> Balzac

An ideal description of health or illness in the child should be concerned not only with symptoms and manifest behaviour, but also with the capacities and adjustments of the child in relation to his maturity, and in the context of the pressures, demands, and supports which he has experienced. Such a description may be made in clinical practice, but inevitably involves inferences beyond directly observable phenomena. For this reason, and because our study was cross-sectional rather than developmental, and because we were assessing the family background as an independent variable, we based our assessment of the children on a standard profile derived from the parents' descriptions.

These parents' descriptions, elicited at interview, were rated against five-point scales, each point on which was illustrated by more or less detailed examples of the type, intensity, and frequency of the attribute being rated. These ratings were a slightly modified version of those developed for the California study carried out by Macfarlane *et al.* (1954); they refer to habit and tension symptoms, on the one hand, and to personality and behavioural items, on the other.

In recording the data for rating these scales, Miss Hamilton did not follow any set order, but the interview was guided to ensure coverage of all the items on the scales. The statements elicited from the parents in this way were recorded in the notes, and ratings were made on them by Miss Hamilton on all the children. Independent rating of a proportion of the case histories by myself showed good agreement, with fewer than one in ten ratings being at variance.

82

These ratings were based upon the child's state over the preceding year. Supplementary data about the children were obtained, both historical (birth, development, separations, etc.) and also a report of any possibly psychosomatic symptoms (these not being included in the Macfarlane ratings). Some inquiry was also made about the child's social participation outside school.

A structured profile of this type is very foreign to psychiatric and casework practice; it did, however, provide a means whereby every child in the population was given an equivalent description which was likely to be moderately free from false generalizations or inferences, either on the part of the parent or on the part of the interviewer. From this profile one could derive both a measure of the amount of disturbance and of its type. The validity of this scoring method was not directly tested in our study. However Brandon (1960), in a study of a sub-sample of the Newcastle 1,000 families, showed that all the 'abnormal' ratings obtained on an abbreviated and modified form of the Macfarlane scales were recorded significantly more often in children independently rated as disturbed. Glidewell *et al.* (1957) have also shown that symptom scores similarly derived from mothers' reports were correlated with independent ratings for disturbance carried out by teachers and psychiatric social workers. The scoring of these rating scales was carried out by allocating scores of 1–3 to those items on each scale which were considered to be 'problem items', this allocation being made on clinical grounds. The classification of 'problem' items followed closely, but not exactly, that used by Macfarlane *et al.* in their original study. In this way a total disturbance score was derived very simply by adding together all those pathological item scores. In addition an arbitrary score of 2 was added where there was a history of recurrent symptomatology suggesting psychosomatic disorder. As well as deriving a total score in this way, we classified the items on clinical grounds into groups as follows: habit and tension symptoms, acting-out behaviour, antisocial behaviour, inhibited behaviour, and compliant social behaviour; there was also a small unclassified group. In this way it was possible to investigate both the distribution of total disturbance scores and the distribution of patterns of disturbance in this child population.

The following two case histories illustrate the type of information rated on these scales.

1. Helen

This was a girl with a high total score on the Macfarlane scales (30) (i.e. in the top 10 percentile), who scored high for inhibited and compliant social behaviour, and for habit and tension symptoms, and low for acting-out and antisocial behaviour. The household consisted of the mother, who was divorced, a maternal aunt some years older than the mother, there being considerable conflict between the mother and this aunt, and Helen, the only child. On the symptom profile Helen was noted to be extremely truthful, although she had truanted from school and had concealed this fact for two weeks; she was over-careful, showed compulsive generosity, and would avoid giving offence at all costs; she was over-sensitive, being upset and over-concerned by family illness or by sad books or television programmes; she was extremely timid and shy with both children and adults and had never in her life lost her temper; she lacked confidence, and she would not compete for fear of failure. The summary description by Miss Hamilton on this child reads as follows:

'Helen is in a conflict of divided loyalties, with increasing insecurity. She is over-identified with mother but openly ambivalent towards the maternal aunt. Like her mother she lacks basic self-esteem, expects rejection from others and is at pains to keep in anyone's good books. At the time of serious rowing between the mother and the maternal aunt, when there was some talk of them separating, Helen developed a "mysterious" skin rash which became generalized, and shortly after this time she truanted from school. Although she had returned to school she had developed an extreme fear of another girl, and going to school has become a real problem. In this, too, she is repeating her mother's pattern, although mother truanted from the senior school. Mother's own health broke down at the time of Helen starting school. With the highly ambivalent relationships within the home the scene seems well set for a possible serious school refusal. Even should this be averted it seems likely that Helen will need direct treatment if she is to become a more effective adult than her mother.'

2. Jack

The family consisted of Jack and two elder brothers. Both parents had grossly deprived childhoods but the marriage was successful. Jack scored a total of 24 on the Macfarlane scales, predominantly on acting-out and antisocial items. Symptom profile reported him as showing a tic, and he was hyper-active, careless, combative, and somewhat selfish. He was unusually unregarding of the feelings of others. In social situations he was entirely confident, and he faced physical risks with bravado. Towards his parents he was often defiant and he had a violent but short-lived temper. He was spontaneous and affectionate. Miss Hamilton's description concluded:

> 'Jack seems to be over-compensating his sense of insecurity with bravado in all fields. At the present moment he is competing fairly successfully with his elder brothers, and also shows a fair amount of dependence on them.'

MACFARLANE SCORES

A detailed statistical study of the scores derived from the Macfarlane scales has been published (Ryle *et al.*, 1965) and it will not be repeated here. It was found that age and sex differences were not marked. In the appendix to this chapter the Macfarlane scales are presented in a highly abbreviated form, and the score allotted to each item is recorded, with the percentage of boys and girls reported at each level being provided. This table serves to emphasize how widespread are 'pathological' symptoms in a 'normal' population. Boys were significantly less timid and shy, and more destructive than girls, and they were more likely to have hearty appetites, but sex differences on the other items were not significant. Total score levels, which are set out in *Table 29*, showed no significant relationship with age or sex. This homogeneity probably reflects the relatively narrow pre-pubertal age range of the sample, and also to some extent the construction of some of the Macfarlane scales, which rate many attributes in relation to the child's age. Sub-group scores for habit and tension symptoms, acting-out and antisocial behaviour and compliant social and inhibited behaviour, also showed no significant

TABLE 29   MACFARLANE SCALES: DISTRIBUTION OF TOTAL
SCORES

Sex	No. assessed	Scores						
		9 or less	10–14	15–19	20–24	25–29	30–34	35 or more
M	79	15	14	15	21	9	3	2
F	80	16	25	15	12	4	3	5

relationship to age or sex. Acting-out, antisocial, and habit and tension symptoms scores were significantly correlated with each other. Inhibited and compliant social scores were correlated with each other and negatively correlated with acting-out and antisocial scores. Children with higher total scores were more likely to show behaviour which was either predominantly acting-out or predominantly inhibited.

One can speculate as to the connection of this division with the congenital differences noted by Chess *et al.* (1960) in their longitudinal study of children from birth. Baldwin's finding (1948) that preschool children with high activity levels showed more non-conformity and rebelliousness when at school is also clearly relevant. How far the much poorer prognosis recorded for acting-out child guidance attenders, reported by O'Neal *et al.* (1958), by Michael *et al.* (1957), and Morris *et al.* (1956) can be considered to apply to this much less disturbed population is uncertain.

The other source of information on the children was the teacher's report. Unfortunately the value of this form is uncertain at this age, the validation study which Douglas and Mulligan (1961) carried out being based upon 13-year-old children. The form consists of a number of questions relating to achievement, behaviour, and personality. Douglas and Mulligan derived a score from this, but their calculations were not completed when we used the instrument, and we therefore relied upon the answers to one of the questions to indicate the teacher's opinion as to the presence and nature of disturbance. This question, No. 23 on the form, reads as follows: 'Taking this child's behaviour and relationships to other children as a whole, would you say he/she is (1) sensitive or highly strung, (2) shy or withdrawn, (3) aggressive, (4) other?', each item being rated 'not at all', 'somewhat', or 'very'. Mulligan had reported (personal communication) that this question did distinguish the child guidance attenders from the controls reasonably satisfactorily. In our sample, where the children were one to six years younger than the children in the validation study, neither the presence of disturbance nor the type, according to the teacher's report, showed any relationship with the total or group scores on the Macfarlane ratings. Educational achievement judged by stream and class position was also unrelated to the Macfarlane scores. It is, of course, likely that the school and home behaviour of children differs sufficiently for a low correlation to be predicted. A study of kindergarten children by Becker (1960), for example, showed low correlations between parents' and teachers' reports.

In the follow-up study it will clearly be of interest to compare the predictive value of the parents' and the school reports upon the children. From the teachers' reports it was also learned that nine boys and one girl were either at special schools or in special classes on account of backwardness.

The ratings and symptom profiles reported above provided the basis for the investigation of family factors associated with disturbance in children and for the discussion of treatment which appears below. They are not adequate, however, to convey the impression given by surveying these 159 children – an impression which is compounded on the one hand of concern at the frequency of behavioural and symptomatic disturbance and at the many and severe family stresses to which the children are exposed, and on the other hand of respect and admiration for the resilience of children and their families. Viewing this sample of children from our various standpoints of general practice, consultant psychiatry, and social work, we differed in detail in our response to these impressions, but were agreed in feeling that a large proportion of the children were liable to be damaged or restricted in their further development, and that therapeutic intervention, had more resources been available, would have been of potential benefit to many families. These impressions were summarized in the form of a 'children's prospects rating' – an overall assessment of the child's chances of attaining maturity and stability – made jointly in the light of the total picture of the family presented by the survey records, taking into account both the child's history and present state and the strengths and problems existing in the family. *Table 30* presents the distribution of the children according to this rating and shows that 28 per cent of the children were considered to have a poor outlook.

TABLE 30   CHILD'S PROSPECTS RATING

Rating	Girls	Boys	Combined
Good or satisfactory	21	13	34 (22%)
Uncertain	37	43	80 (50%)
Poor or very poor	22	23	45 (28%)

This chapter has been concerned with psychological symptoms; to balance this account it should be recorded that chronic physical ill health was virtually absent (although one child had been excluded on account of a potentially fatal condition). Four children, however, were epileptic, three of whom required medication, and six others had had febrile convulsions. Three children had had asthma, one moderately severely. One child had to attend a special school on account of poor vision. Beyond this, physical illness consisted of the usual and inevitable infections, of which the only known permanent sequelae were two chronically perforated eardrums. Contrasting this record with the figures for psychological disturbance, one is forced to ask whether the shift in emphasis in the medical and social services towards giving attention to psychiatric problems is proceeding with adequate speed.

APPENDIX TO CHAPTER 7

Habit and tension symptoms scale

Scale title (Macfarlane equivalent in brackets)	Abbreviated description	Score	Percentage distribution	
			Boys	Girls
Restless sleep (A. 1 and 2 combined)	1. 2 hours or more delay and/or walks, talks, cries most nights.	3	30	23
	2. Often delayed; talks, walks or very restless weekly or more.	2	14	10
	3. Disturbed weekly to monthly.	1	6	16
	4. Rarely delayed or disturbed.	0	16	16
	5. Usually sound quiet sleeper.	0	34	35
Nocturnal enuresis (B.4)	1. Wet 2 or more times weekly.	3	4	6
	2. 2–7 times monthly.	2	0	3
	3. Monthly.	1	5	3
	4. Once in past six months.	0	10	7
	5. Not in past six months.	0	81	81
Appetite (C.7)	1. Markedly poor.	3	4	6
	2. Below average.	1	18	40
	3. Average.	0	29	29
	4. Hearty appetite.	0	32	22
	5. Voracious.	2	17	3
Motor habits (E.15, 18, 19 combined)	1. Tics, nail-biting, thumb-sucking Compulsive, severe, persistent.	3	4	6
	2. Obvious and usually present.	2	19	18
	3. Mild and/or only under tension.	1	24	26
	4. Mild, infrequent, irregular habits.	0	18	18
	5. Absent.	0	35	32

Neurosis in the Ordinary Family

Activity level (at home) (E.20)				
	1. Restless always; very over-active.	3	1	3
	2. More restless than average.	2	33	23
	3. Normal activity.	0	56	64
	4. Under-active, prefers sedentary occupations.	0	9	10
	5. Inert, inactive.	0	1	0

Acting-out (AO) and inhibited (I) scales

Scale title (Macfarlane equivalent in brackets)	Abbreviated description	Score	Sub-group	Percentage distribution Boys	Girls
Destructive-ness (F.24 modified)	1. Compulsive.	3	AO	0	0
	2. Above average. Very clumsy.	2	AO	19	10
	3. Occasionally careless or destructive through curiosity.	0	—	68	55
	4. Very careful but able to enjoy playing nonetheless.	0	—	12	27
	5. Excessive care inhibits enjoyment.	3	I	1	8
Selfishness (F.26 modified)	1. Strongly resents sharing.	3	AO	1	1
	2. Shares under pressure; thoughtless.	2	AO	24	13
	3. Normally will share happily except favourite toys.	0	—	34	39
	4. Enjoys sharing and giving presents.	0	—	27	37
	5. Over-generous; inhibited by fear of troubling others.	3	I	14	10

Quarrelsome-	1. Constant quarrelling.	3	AO	1	0
ness	2. Above average quarrelling.	2	AO	4	1
(F.27)	3. Quarrels with provocation, may occasionally start.	0	—	52	35
	4. Below average quarrelling.	0	—	29	43
	5. Compulsive placation.	3	I	14	21

Demanding	1. Constant demand for attention.	3	AO	5	5
(G.29 modified)	2. Above average demand for attention.	2	AO	38	46
	3. Likes attention but functions without it.	0	—	35	34
	4. Usually quite content without attention.	0	—	18	11
	5. Unusually self-contained and self-reliant.	2	I	4	4

Timidity	1. Fearful, apprehensive.	3	I	3	5
(G.36)	2. Over-cautious.	1	I	11	20
	3. Normally cautious.	0	—	27	35
	4. Exploratory, will take chances.	0	—	46	35
	5. Foolhardy.	2	AO	13	5

Shyness	1. Exceptionally shy.	3	I	0	0
(G.36b modified)	2. Often shy, embarrassed in company.	2	I	37	20
	3. Shy with certain people only.	0	—	38	51
	4. At ease in most social situations.	0	—	8	19
	5. Facile contacts.	2	AO	17	10

91

Defiance (G.40)	1. Extreme, pervasive negativism.	3	AO	0	1
	2. Above average resistiveness.	2	AO	27	21
	3. Occasionally resistive, especially of unreasonable demands.	0	—	66	58
	4. Accepts rules and routines automatically.	0	—	6	17
	5. Docile, over-suggestible.	3	I	1	3

Scored on severity × frequency

Temper tantrums (G.42)	1. Severe, over 3 weekly.	3	AO	17	6
	2. Occasionally severe; frequent screaming.	2	AO	16	14
	3. Less severe than in 2.	1	AO	35	34
	4. Minor fretting when irritated.	0	—	16	22
	5. Over-placid, almost no anger reaction.	3	I	16	24

Jealousy (G.43)	1. Extreme. Overt.	3	AO	4	3
	2. Less extreme; constant.	2	AO	18	24
	3. Occasional; mild.	1	AO	25	29
	4. No real jealousy; occasionally needs reassurance.	0	—	50	33
	5. No jealousy.	0	—	3	11

Competitiveness (G.44 modified)	1. Hectic. Extreme.	3	AO	0	1
	2. Hates losing, excessively cocky if wins.	2	AO	1	0
	3. Stimulated by competition, can accept defeat.	0	—	28	23
	4. Not competitive.	0	—	70	70
	5. Fails compulsively or through disorganization.	3	I	1	6

Reserve (G.45)	1. Extreme reserve.	3	I	4	0
	2. Above average reserve.	2	I	33	25
	3. Normally expressive.	0	—	39	50
	4. Spontaneous, open, volatile.	0	—	23	20
	5. Very uninhibited. Exhibitionistic.	2	AO	1	5

Antisocial (AS) and compliant social (CS) scales

Scale title (Macfarlane equivalent in brackets)	Abbreviated description	Score	Sub-group	Percentage distribution Boys	Girls
Lying (F.22)	1. Habitual. Compulsive.	3	AS	0	1
	2. Above average.	2	AS	9	10
	3. Occasional.	1	AS	43	24
	4. Never or only under stress.	0	—	38	56
	5. Never, regardless of consequences.	2	CS	10	9
Truancy (from home or school) (F.22a, 22b combined)	1. Wanders more than weekly.	3	AS	5	1
	2. Weekly to monthly wandering.	2	AS	6	1
	3. Monthly wandering.	1	AS	19	15
	4. Occasionally fails to say, or late back.	0	—	61	64
	5. Home-tied. Never late or out without permission.	2	CS	9	19
Stealing (F.23)	1. Persistent, compulsive, including valuables.	3	AS	0	0
	2. Chronic petty pilfering, home or outside.	2	AS	3	4
	3. Occasional pilfering outside home, money from parents.	1	AS	10	3
	4. Occasional 'borrowing'.	0	—	46	42
	5. Never steals; looks for owner if finds lost property.	1	CS	41	51

Unclassified scales

Scale title (Macfarlane equivalent in brackets)	Abbreviated description	Score	Percentage distribution	
			Boys	Girls
Sensitive	1. Super-sensitive.	3	4	5
(G.35)	2. Over-sensitive.	2	41	44
	3. Normally responsive.	0	35	35
	4. Matter-of-fact, not easily hurt or upset.	0	15	13
	5. Callous, indifferent.	3	5	3
Specific fears	1. Extreme, incapacitating.	3	3	0
(G.37	2. Less extreme; may lead to flight.	3	6	8
modified)	3. Certain marked fears (e.g. dark, dogs).	2	19	24
	4. Slight apprehension; can face in company.	1	38	24
	5. No fears beyond legitimate caution.	0	34	44
Lack of confidence	1. Parents' approval dominates values and interests.	3	1	1
(G.46 modified consider-ably)	2. Needs constant approval; easily swayed.	2	27	23
	3. Likes to try alone, may need reassurance.	0	37	50
	4. Prefers not to be helped.	0	33	23
	5. Rejects assistance, aggressively independent.	2	2	3

CHAPTER 8

Parental Factors associated with
Disturbance in the Children

'John is in such spirits today!' said she, on his taking Miss
Steeles' pocket handkerchief and throwing it out of the win-
dow – 'he is full of monkey tricks.' And soon afterwards, on
the second boy's violently pinching one of the same lady's
fingers, she fondly observed 'How playful William is!'

Jane Austen, *Sense and sensibility*

A large number of ratings of various aspects of family functioning
have been reported in previous chapters. Many of these refer to
factors likely to be relevant to the presence or absence of disturbance
in the child. These factors are complex, and the measures made of
them are of varying validity and reliability. In some cases they have
been shown to be interrelated, for example parents' childhood,
marital rating, and child-rearing behaviour, while in other cases
predicted relationships do not appear, for example interview and
inventory ratings of parental behaviour.

We were forced to reduce the number of factors investigated
statistically to a manageable number, and decided to restrict the
main statistical analysis to those variables referring directly to one
or other parent. The measures of disturbance in the children, i.e. the
outcome variables, were: (1) The Macfarlane scores of the children,
and (2) The teachers' reports on the children. The former were presented as total scores, as acting-out anti-social combined scores (AO
+AS), and as inhibited/compliant-social combined scores (I+CS).
The teachers' reports (see Chapter 7) were presented as showing no
disturbance, acting-out behaviour (rated 'very aggressive' by teacher),
or inhibited behaviour (rated 'very sensitive' or 'very shy').

The parental variables, which form the basis of the statistical
study, are summarized below:

1. Variables referring to the mother:

(a) Childhood adversity was scored 1–6 according to the scale position on the rating described for childhood experience in Chapter 6.

(b) The presence or absence of minimal neurosis as defined in Chapter 4.

(c) Interview ratings of parental behaviour (see Chapter 6) as follows:

—Neurotic involvement rated as absent (0), present (1), or marked (2).

—Consistency rated 1–5 on the scale given in the appendix to Chapter 6.

—Acceptance rated by summing scores on five scales as described in the appendix to Chapter 6.

—Domination. This was rated by summing scores from the scales for discipline, esteem building, and over-protection (see Chapter 6). This procedure was later seen to be dubious, but by this time the data were already in the computer. It was found, on a sample of 59 parents, that the parent discipline rating correlated with the sum of the scores on the other two ratings at a level of $r = 0.3$ only. High scores on this combined domination measure therefore represent an uncertain mixture of strict discipline, over-protection, and undermining. This domination measure was presented in two forms: (i) as a straight domination score, and (ii) as a measure of high or low domination, intermediate scores getting 0, and high or low scores (called for brevity 'extremes of domination') getting 1. This latter procedure was based on the assumption that extremes of domination, whether high or low, were likely to be harmful to the child.

(d) Inventory ratings of parental behaviour. These were derived from the inventory described in Chapter 6. The acceptance and domination scores were used direct; the latter was also presented as intermediate = 0, high or low ('extremes of domination') = 1, as was the case with the interview ratings.

2. Variables referring to the father. The same range of factors was rated for the fathers, except that no inventory rating of acceptance was available, and the inventory domination score was reduced to a 3-point rating, owing to the fact that two different versions of the instrument had been used.

Parental Factors associated with Disturbance in the Children

3. Separation and substitutions:

(a) Separation from both parents away from home before the age of five was rated as nil (score 0); less than one month (score 1) (this was experienced by 38 children); and more than one month (score 2) (experienced by 46 children).

(b) Parent substitution by another significant adult was rated as none (0), present (1), and present and of critical importance (2).

STATISTICAL PROCEDURE

The main statistical study was carried out upon 69 boys and 69 girls on whom the full range of data was available and who had two parents. The conventional statistical method for this type of study would probably be factor analysis, but there are theoretical objections to this approach (see for example Dahlstrom, 1957). In our study, where both the background and child variables were rated by the same observer, the possibility of extracting factors that represent no more than the patterns of preconceptions already held seemed considerable. We therefore adopted the alternative approach of multiple regressions. By this method, the relation of each background factor to the children's scores could be examined while allowing for the effects of all the other factors. This method also guards against distortions which might arise from the inclusion of invalid measures. This statistical procedure was carried out for us by Miss Ruth Tall (M.R.C. Statistical Research Unit), and the programming was done by Miss Margaret Devine, to both of whom we are very grateful. The details of this will be published elsewhere and are not reproduced here in full. The main results are summarized below, in *Table 31*.

This table summarizes the significant associations found between the parental factors, the various Macfarlane scores, and the teachers' classification, recording the level of significance of the association found and the percentage of total variance accounted for by the factors. In a table of this size some chance correlations would be expected, but the significance levels of those reported suggest that the relationships indicated are genuine. In summary, these are as follows: the reservations about the interview domination measure should be borne in mind.

TABLE 31 SUMMARY OF ASSOCIATIONS FOUND BY MULTIPLE REGRESSIONS OF PARENTAL FACTORS ON CHILDREN'S MACFARLANE SCORES AND TEACHERS' CLASSIFICATION

Parental factor	Child's Macfarlane Score						Teacher's classification			
	Boys			Girls			Boys		Girls	
	Total	AO+AS	I+CS	Total	AO+AS	I+CS	Aggressive	Inhibited	Aggressive	Inhibited
(a) Mother										
Childhood adversity										
Minimal neurosis						+				
Child-rearing (Int. rating)										
Low consistency	++	++								
Neurotic involvement	++	++	++		+		+			
High domination		−								
Extremes of domination				+	+					
High acceptance		−								
Child-rearing (Inv. rating)										
High domination						−				
Extremes of domination		+								
High acceptance				−	−					
(b) Father										
Childhood adversity						−		−		
Minimal neurosis						+				
Child-rearing (Int. rating)										
Low consistency										
Neurotic involvement						+				
High domination										
Extremes of domination		+							+	
High acceptance										
Child-rearing (Inv. rating)										
High domination								+		
Extremes of domination										
(c) Deprivation & substitution										
Separation experience		−								
Significant parental substitutes										
p level of association	<0·001	÷0·002	÷0·005	÷0·025	÷0·015	÷0·002	÷0·025	÷0·01	÷0·005	
% of variance accounted for	32	28	13	11	15	29	7	13	11	

Parental Factors associated with Disturbance in the Children

Maternal factors and disturbance in boys
Sons of neurotically involved mothers tended to have high total, AO+AS, and I+CS scores and they tended to be noted as aggressive at school. Inconsistency in the mother was also associated with high total and AO+AS scores. Highly accepting mothers tended to have sons with low AO+AS scores. Mothers who were themselves minimally neurotic were less likely to bring their sons to consult for psychological difficulties. High domination (interview rating) was associated with low AO+AS scores and high I+CS scores.

Maternal factors and disturbance in girls
Daughters whose mothers were neurotically involved tended to have high AO+AS scores. Extremes of domination (interview assessment) were associated with high total and AO+AS scores. High domination (inventory measure) was associated with low I+CS scores. Mothers who were themselves minimally neurotic tended to have daughters with high I+CS scores.

Paternal factors and disturbance in boys
Only three significant associations were found. Extremes of domination (inventory rating) were associated with a teacher's rating of the boy as inhibited, whereas extremes of domination (interview rating) were associated with high AO+AS scores. Fathers who had themselves had adverse childhood experience were unlikely to have their sons rated by teachers as inhibited.

Paternal factors and disturbance in girls
Fathers who were rated high for acceptance tended to have daughters with low total and AO+AS scores. Daughters of neurotically involved fathers tended to have high I+CS scores, and the same applied where the father was minimally neurotic. Fathers who had experienced adverse childhood tended to have daughters with low I+CS scores. Fathers rated as showing extremes of domination (interview rating) tended to have daughters classified by the teachers as aggressive.

It will be noted from this table that more maternal than paternal factors show significant associations with the Macfarlane scores of the children, and that more associations of parental factors are found with the scores of children of opposite sex.

99

PARENTS' MARITAL ADJUSTMENT AND LOSS OF PARENTS

Among factors not included in the above statistical analysis, two are worthy of note: the parents' marital adjustment, and the absence, for whatever reason, of one or other parent. It was found that the total Macfarlane scores were significantly lower in the case of girls where the parents' marriage was well rated (1 or 2) ($\chi^2 = 4.6$, $p < 0.05$); but there was no association with boys' scores. Of 17 children from 13 one-parent homes (in all but two the father being absent), only five scored 20 or more on the Macfarlane scales, a proportion lower than was the case in the population as a whole.

DISCUSSION

The fact that a relatively small proportion of the total variance in the children's scores was accounted for by the range of parental factors studied is not entirely surprising. Clearly, genetic factors must account for some of the remaining variation, even if, as Rutter *et al.* (1964) have argued, symptomatology is only evoked when genetic and environmental factors interact. Without doubt, also, the crudity of the rating methods of both parent and child variables may be expected to minimize some associations.

Beyond this one must consider the assumptions underlying the correlating of background factors with symptom and behaviour scores. In this approach one is, by implication, assuming that all children are likely to respond to a certain form of parental behaviour in a similar way and that all instances of a certain form of behaviour in children are likely to be the consequence of the same parental factors. One does not need to know more than two children to realize that this assumption requires considerable qualification. The demonstration of any correlations between background factors and children's behaviour and symptoms could therefore be regarded as gratifying. One is showing that a given class of parental behaviour, despite the variations within it, despite the different ways in which different children will construe it, and despite the different learned and genetically-determined patterns of response available to the children, tends to be associated with a particular pattern of behaviour or symptoms in children.

The meaning placed upon the associations demonstrated must

depend in part upon the validity and reliability of the measures used. In view of the major methodological weaknesses of our interview domination rating, mentioned above, not much weight should be placed upon this factor; while there is little doubt that extreme scores on this scale indicate adverse parental behaviour, the nature of this behaviour is not clearly defined. The measures of parental neuroticism, and the interview measures of consistency and acceptance, are probably reasonably valid. The rating of parental neurotic involvement with the child – the factor with most frequent associations with the children's scores – is a clinical one made jointly by A.R. and M.H., and the possibility of interviewer bias must be acknowledged. We were, however, very much aware of this danger, and every attempt was made to base this rating on the parents' descriptions of their attitudes and behaviour and upon their behaviour at interview, and not upon global impressions or hunches. The fact that only one inventory measure of parental attitudes was significantly associated with the children's scores would tend to underline the reservations expressed about these instruments in Chapter 6.

The associations which have been demonstrated are largely in line with those found by others. The association of high maternal domination with inhibited behaviour in boys agrees with Baldwin's study (1948) and with the 'repressive over-control' group in the study by Hewitt and Jenkins (1946). Maternal inconsistency has been related to acting-out antisocial behaviour by Rosenthal (1962). Acting-out behaviour is associated in our study with low acceptance by the opposite-sex parent and, in the case of boys, with non-dominant mothers, a finding in line with the delinquent 'unsocialized aggression' group in the study by Hewitt and Jenkins, and with the aggressive in-patient group studied by Morris *et al.* (1956). Neuroticism in both fathers and mothers was associated only with inhibited behaviour in girls; this finding, and the fact that the girls' total Macfarlane scores, but not those of the boys, were related to the marital rating, are of some interest. It will be recalled (Chapter 4) that mothers remembered more emotional disturbance in their childhood homes than did the fathers, and that the association of this recall with neuroticism was significant only in the case of mothers.

As regards the direction of the associations demonstrated, those between high domination and inhibition, and between low domination and acting-out behaviour, seem likely to be causal from parent

101

to child, since inhibited behaviour in the child would hardly provoke parental strictness, and acting-out behaviour would hardly provoke laxness. Parental childhood experience and parental neuroticism are two other factors likely to have preceded the birth of the child, and therefore the relationship with children's scores is likely to be causal from parent to child also. Neurotic involvement, as defined, is related to the parents' own psychodynamics, but becomes of course a mutual affair between parent and child. Low consistency, low acceptance, and extremes of domination in parents could conceivably be either causal of acting-out/antisocial behaviour or reactive to it. The negative association of separation experience with acting-out and antisocial behaviour is contrary to the assumption often held, although it should be noted that neither Andry (1960) nor Lewis (1954) found any specific link between parental deprivation and delinquency.

In summary, the associations between the behaviour, attitudes, and personality of parents and the psychological disturbance of their children that have been demonstrated are largely in line with associations found in other studies of different types of population. This can be taken as further evidence for an important environmental contribution to the genesis of such disturbance. The relative importance of nature and nurture remains uncertain, however. The relatively small proportion of variance accounted for by the factors included in our study can probably be attributed to the restricted range of factors included, to deficiencies in the methods of measurement used, and to the unsubtle nature of the associations tested.

CHAPTER 9

Family Diagnosis

It is clear that organized study of the area of the family and mental illness is in a state of chaos.

J. H. Cumming (1961)

Although this is a book about families, with the exception of the statistical study in the last chapter it has been concerned with only parts of the family, focusing on individuals, on the parental pair in the marriage relationship, on parent–child interaction, or on the child's symptoms. This is no accident, for the conceptual problems of studying total family functioning are considerable even at a purely descriptive level, and our research, while providing some quantitative and some illustrative data, was neither based upon, nor aiming to test, any theoretical model of family functioning.

In the present chapter I shall discuss, without any pretensions to special competence or to a comprehensive knowledge of the field, aspects of family diagnosis of possible clinical use; it should be emphasized that this does not set out to meet the rigorous demands of a testable theoretical system, and I am only too aware that it is still diffuse and unsatisfactory. There are many sources from which I have drawn, and by which I have been influenced; many of these are referred to below, others include: Rogers (1951); Mowrer, (1950, 1953); Spiegel and Bell (1959); Dicks (1959); Tharp (1963), and Cumming (1961), whose gloomy comment on his own review of the field, quoted above, may mitigate the reader's judgement of this chapter.

For doctors and social workers, a family diagnosis must be primarily concerned with those aspects of family functioning related to the stabilization or exacerbation of the psychological state of the members of the family, and must take into account the following areas (arranged in this list more or less in order of increasing clinical relevance):

1. The family in relation to society.
2. The family in relation to the extended family.
3. The relation between sickness in different family members.
4. The diagnosis of family relationships.

In the rest of this chapter I shall attempt to examine these areas in turn, providing some examples from the research records. As explained in the introduction, the reproduction of detailed individual family case histories was considered unjustifiable; as a poor second best I shall illustrate each aspect of family diagnosis with two examples from the research case records giving the family composition, the main ratings applied to various aspects of the family, and the relevant diagnostic formulation. The following ratings will be included:

1. The parents' social participation rating (described in Chapter 2).
2. The children's social participation rating.
3. The mothers' household management rating.
4. The family unity rating.
5. The children's prospects rating.

The scales for these last four ratings are provided in the appendix to this chapter.

1. THE FAMILY IN RELATION TO SOCIETY

The two central functions of the family, according to Parsons and Bales (1955), are to provide for the stabilization of the parents and the socialization of children. Because the forms through which these functions are fulfilled (and the economic importance of the family in society) show major differences between different cultures and classes, research into the role of the family in psychological illness cannot ignore the social and cultural setting of family groups studied, and therapy must be based upon understanding of these factors. Moreover this is an area of family functioning which is immediately relevant to much casework and medical practice, even in relatively stable and affluent Western societies. On the one hand there are the socially deviant families who absorb a large part of social work effort, in which major and multiple pressures and deprivations operate and where psychiatric disorder may be seen both as one result and one cause of the family's social breakdown. This type of family has been described by recent books such as Harriet Wilson's *Delinquency and child neglect* (1962), and Philp's *Family failure* (1963). In our survey population severe social pressures and relative economic hardship were most apparent in those families in which children were being reared by a mother without the help of a father. Apart from social breakdown, or dependency, there are commoner, less gross forms of social maladaptation of relevance to psychiatry, both as causes and as results of psychological abnormality. These include antisocial behaviour (criminality or delinquency), low job stability, and the whole range of eccentric, mildly deviant, or non-conformist behaviours which grade imperceptibly into the normal range. With these, one needs to bear in mind the point of view of writers such as Fromm (1961) who argue that to some extent conformity to our society may be a sign of, or achieved only at the cost of, some restriction of personality.

The other way in which the family's cultural and social setting is of relevance to the professional worker is in respect of the barrier to communication set up by cultural and class differences both in terms of language and of underlying assumptions. Hollingshead and Redlich (1958) have shown how class similarity influences selection of patients for psychotherapy, and Carstairs (1958), writing of patients from alien cultures, has argued that in some ways the working-class sub-culture is sufficiently alien to that of most psychiatrists to constitute a block to communication. It could be argued that cultural factors were often just as important as those imposed by the professional worker's personality difficulties, although this is an area which, in comparison with the therapist's personality, has been very little studied. Social distance certainly influences the acceptability or otherwise of casework help, and the social worker, possibly owing to her historical roots in charity and 'do-gooding', has an image which is by no means unblemished in the public eye. Hoggart (1958) in *The uses of literacy* mentions how the family doctor seems to be the best-accepted middle-class individual in working-class communities, perhaps because his role is clearly defined – an observation that might perhaps be taken as providing some support for the suggestion that general practice would be a satisfactory base for family casework.

In summary, therefore, the formulation of a family diagnosis must take into account both the manifest adjustment of the family to its society and the underlying cultural values to which its members adhere. Family treatment must aim to overcome the social barriers between the patient or client and the doctor or caseworker.

Family diagnosis illustrations – the family in relation to society

(*i*) The Carter family
Family composition: Mother aged 49; William (son of her broken marriage, now in Australia); three illegitimate children: James aged 10, Arthur aged nine, David aged seven; putative father visits regularly and provides maintenance.

Family ratings (figures in brackets refer to placing on appropriate scales): Mother came from an intact home with major emotional disturbance (5), was neurotic (C.M.I. score 39), and the marriage was broken (5). The three children scored in the lower ranges on the Macfarlane scales (9, 11, and 7). Mother was socially isolated, without support (1), but managed the household efficiently (2). The children had several friends (2), and the family was united (1). Mother was adequately accepting, intermediate on the domination scale, did not show neurotic involvement with the children. The children's prospects were rated as uncertain (3).

Diagnostic formulation (in relation to society): This was a family with a psychiatrically disturbed, illiterate, socially isolated mother, with three illegitimate sons who showed no evidence of disturbance except for poor school achievement. The relation of this family to society can be described as one of social deviance, isolation, and relative privation. The mother suffered from depression and paranoid feelings, which at times had reached psychotic intensity, that could be seen as both one reflection and as one cause of her relation to society.

(*ii*) The Able family
Family composition: Paternal grandfather aged 72; father aged 53, a coachdriver; mother aged 47, a telephonist; a son away in the merchant navy; Michael aged 14; Jill aged 11.

Family ratings: Father came from an intact home with major emotional disturbance (5), mother from an emotionally secure intact home (1). Both parents were neurotic (C.M.I. of both was 40). There was open conflict in the marriage (4), with both partners showing unmet dependent needs, the father dominating. Jill scored in the upper range on the Macfarlane ratings (23). Only the father had any social participation outside the home (3). Jill had several friends, however (2). The family showed major differences and disunity (3), but mother was an efficient manager of the household (2). Father was consistent but rigid; high domination, low acceptance. Mother was variable in consistency; low domination, low acceptance, and she was considered to show marked neurotic involvement. Jill's prospects were regarded as poor (4).

Diagnostic formulation (in relation to society): This was a family with many emotional stresses in which all members had overt psychological symptoms, where the social manifestations of the disturbance were less obvious than in the case of the Carter family. Economic standards were high and both parents had good work records. The father was the only member of the family with meaningful contacts outside the home, being active in various community affairs; to some extent these activities could be seen as the expression of his own internal drives but, even though making a real contribution, he felt unfulfilled in this sphere also. Mother's unhappiness and dissatisfactions had been expressed by frequent (twice successful) demands for rehousing on the basis of noisy neighbours. Jill had shown antisocial behaviour by truanting and by misbehaviour at school.

2. THE FAMILY IN RELATION TO THE EXTENDED FAMILY

As Young and Willmott (1962) have demonstrated, the working-class nuclear family is by no means isolated from the network of relatives, even if social changes now occurring may be tending to weaken the links. In our own study we found a degree of contact with the extended family of the same order as that described in Bethnal Green by these writers. The nature of this was variable and the reasons for contact or non-contact were themselves psychologically important. Hence no clear relationship could be demonstrated between the degree of contact with the extended family and the psychological state of the family members. Theoretically one could see that both a continued close relationship of the parents with the grandparents (possibly implying unresolved dependence) and rupture of the relationship (possibly implying previous major conflict) might be related to neurosis in the parents. More generally, one might predict that acceptance by the extended family and continued social activity within it might well have a stabilizing effect, but one might also see how the ability to enlarge and choose one's own social circle might be evidence of maturity and of a more positive adaptation to society as a whole. From the point of view of research, therefore, this is a complex problem to investigate; from the point of view of treatment it is quite clear that the significant others in the neurotic patient's world may well include not only members of the nuclear family but also members of the extended family, with grandparents providing the most frequent significant figures.

Family diagnosis illustrations – the family in relation to the extended family

(i) The Wake family
Family composition: Father, a decorator, aged 30; mother aged 27; Kenneth aged eight; Ronald aged seven. The maternal grandmother lived a few doors away, and was in the house every day.
Family ratings: Father came from an intact home with minor emotional disturbance (4): mother had lost her father in childhood but had had secure care from the mother (3). Mother scored 20 on the C.M.I., father 11, neither therefore falling within the neurotic range. The marital rating was 3 (stresses contained), the wife being considered dominating and having immature, unmet dependent needs. Of the children both scored in the top range of the Macfarlane scales (Kenneth 38, Ronald 25); Kenneth was solitary (5), whereas Ronald had several friends (2). The parents' social participation was confined to the extended family (3); mother was an efficient household manager (2), but the family was disunited (3). Mother was totally inconsistent, gave low acceptance, low domination, and had marked neurotic involvement with the children; father was consistent and flexible (1), but low in acceptance, intermediate on domination, and was considered also to show some neurotic involvement. Kenneth was considered to have a poor outlook (4), Ronald uncertain (3).

Diagnostic formulation (related to extended family): This was a family with a neurotic mother and with disturbance in both children; Ronald (who was, incidentally, the less disturbed) having been referred for child guidance. The maternal grandmother was an important, largely negative influence. The family was intensely involved with her: she both dominated the mother and was in alliance with her in her undermining of the husband and in her rejection and scapegoating of Kenneth. Thus both the marital relationship and the child-rearing practices of the couple were influenced by the maternal grandmother's intervention.

(ii) The Lancaster family

Family composition: Father, a draughtsman, aged 30; mother aged 29; Evelyn aged eight; Edward aged seven.

Family ratings: Both the parents of this family came from intact homes in which there had been major emotional disturbance (5), and both were in the probable neurotic range in the C.M.I. scores (mother 64, father 25). The marriage was rated as 3 (stresses contained), the husband being dominating and the wife having unmet dependent needs. The children scored within the normal range on the Macfarlane scales (Evelyn 5, Edward 19). This was an isolated family with no social participation (1), although the children were active club members (1). Mother was an efficient and flexible housewife (2). The family was considered to show minor differences (2). As regards child-rearing, the father showed variable consistency, intermediate domination, and low acceptance; the mother showed variable consistency, intermediate domination, and adequate acceptance. The prospects of both children were considered poor (4).

Diagnostic formulation (related to extended family): This was a family where the father's dominating behaviour towards his wife was seen as damaging to the wife and to the children. This behaviour originated in his own relationship with his parents, both in their rejection of him in childhood and in their opposition to his marriage and rejection of his wife. The family had a positive and potentially dependent relationship with the extended family on the mother's side, but none of them lived within 200 miles. Since before the marriage the wife had been excluded from all contact with the husband's family; the husband had remained ambivalently involved with his parents, angered by their behaviour but, at least in the early years of

109

the marriage, attempting to placate them, often at the cost of neglecting his wife. Later, contact with his family had been progressively reduced. These parents were therefore very isolated but they had shown some ability to grow in maturity and mutual understanding over the years of their marriage.

3. THE RELATION BETWEEN SICKNESS IN DIFFERENT FAMILY MEMBERS

In medical practice one normally encounters only those patients who have chosen to consult with symptoms. The family-centred caseworker or doctor, however, cannot take symptoms or consultation as an index of illness: he must take into account the behaviour, relationships, maturity, and the development of potential of each individual. Whitehorn (1962) provides a useful and simple framework for the assessment of maturity in his paper 'A working concept of maturity of personality'. He relates the growth of maturity to three basic emotional needs: the need for affection, the need for personal security, and the need for personal significance. Having discussed the development of the ways in which these needs are satisfied through childhood and adolescence, he concludes:

'... complete maturity is an ideal and only approximated in reality. In what we call the mature personality a manageable flexibility of social attitudes has been achieved; this is manifested in a variety of role behaviours developed through life experiences which have served to fulfil emotional needs reasonably well. The mature individual has not graduated to a stage in which he no longer has these needs, rather he has attained flexibility in accepting and acting out the roles which satisfy these emotional needs.'

In the case of children, an adequate criterion of health must include an assessment of the degree to which the successive phases or crises of development are accomplished. Erikson (1950) has contributed to this field by forging a link between psycho-analysis and an awareness of social forces. Epstein (1958), developing his argument from Erikson and others, puts forward a working classification which he has used for research purposes: it is based upon symptomatology, the degree of social and occupational adaptation, and the degree of 'dynamic integration'. In his assessment of dynamic integration,

110

Epstein looks for 'a satisfactory resolution of all the intra- and extra-psychic adaptive problems which should have been dealt with by the individual in his development up to the point of his examination'. One can see that this very interpretative measure would raise considerable problems of method in a research programme, but it is a useful approach in the clinical description of a family situation.

The following case histories show how the family members who are central to the family disturbance are not necessarily the ones to present in consultation.

Family diagnosis illustrations – the relation between sickness in different family members

(*i*) *The Fox family*
Family composition: Father, an engineer, aged 45; mother aged 45; Jonathan aged 17; survey child Elaine aged 10. The paternal grandmother lived next door.
Family ratings: The father came from an intact home where there had been major emotional disturbance (5); mother came from an intact and emotionally secure home (1). Mother's C.M.I. score was 25, father's 23. The marriage was rated 3 (stresses contained), the husband being seen as dominating. Elaine's Macfarlane score was in the upper range (23). The parents' social participation was confined to the extended family (2), as was the child's (3). Mother was a not very efficient housewife (4), and the family was seen as fragmented (4). Mother's consistency was variable (3), acceptance low, domination intermediate, neurotic involvement present; father's consistency was high (1), acceptance adequate, domination low. Neurotic involvement marked. Elaine's prospects were rated as poor (4).
Diagnostic formulation (illness in the family): This was a family in which only one member, the father, had presented with symptoms, but the personalities and relationships of all members were probably markedly deviant. Mother, while never consulting, was an isolated, restricted person, coping with the practical management of the house but perplexed by, although on the whole accepting of, the father and the son. The father, who had seen a psychiatrist twelve years previously, but had had no treatment since, appeared to be an abnormal, schizoid personality, as was Jonathan who had never been able to get over his rivalry with, and jealousy of, Elaine, and who still played

111

with children four or five years his junior. Elaine herself showed overt evidence of psychological disturbance both at home and at school, with isolation, dependence upon private fantasy games, and a preoccupation with occult matters and religious symbolism which she shared with her father.

(ii) The Wolf family

Family composition: Father aged 40, a shopkeeper; mother aged 39; Jean aged 12; Pamela aged six.

Family ratings: Both parents came from intact homes with minor emotional disturbances (4). Mother scored 19 and father 16 on the C.M.I. The marriage was rated as stresses contained (3), with the husband dominating. Jean scored in the upper range on the Macfarlane scales (23), Pamela scored 12. The parents showed some social contacts (3), and Jean was active in clubs (1) but Pamela was confined to family contacts only (3). Mother was a moderately efficient housewife (3). Family unity was rated as poor (3). Mother's consistency was variable (3), acceptance low, domination intermediate; father's consistency was low, acceptance low, domination high. Both parents showed neurotic involvement with Jean, whose prospects were rated as poor (4); Pamela's prospects were rated uncertain (3).

Diagnostic formulation (illness in the family): This was a family with a driving, ambitious father, a depressed, placatory mother, and two psychologically disturbed children. Mother had had a severe depression during her pregnancy with Pamela and had wished to have the child adopted; Pamela had slept at home, but had been reared largely by a foster-parent. Both the children had given direct evidence of psychological disturbance, Jean in jealousy, defiance, and withdrawal, Pamela in enuresis; only the latter had been brought to consultation. The main source of stress in the family, however, was the father, whose freedom from psychological 'illness' had been achieved at the cost of the neglect of his own physical health (he had tuberculosis and had failed to follow advice or remain under supervision) and of his family's psychological health. This was due to his intense, driving ambition to establish himself in business. It seemed possible that the family would survive as a unit and be less stress-ridden if father in fact succeeded in achieving his aim, because there were apparently still positive aspects to the relationship between the parents.

112

4. THE DIAGNOSIS OF RELATIONSHIPS

(*a*) *Dimensions of interpersonal behaviour*

Research workers in the field both of child-rearing practices and of marital interaction have described interaction in terms of two major dimensions, namely *acceptance–rejection* and *domination–submission* (e.g. Winch, 1958; Schaefer, 1961; Roe and Siegelman, 1963). Acceptance refers to co-operation, working together, helping, nurturing, and loving; and domination refers to controlling, coercing, possessing, dominating, and undermining. The definition of domination applied to the marital relationship in Chapter 5 provides a distinction between domination and leadership. Where leadership towards an agreed goal is accepted, it can better be regarded as a special form of co-operation – a distinction that is often ignored. For example, the absolute control exercised by the captain of a ship, or by a surgeon in the operating theatre, is a necessary feature of the enterprise and is accepted by the crew, or by the theatre staff, in the interests of the ship or of the patient. However, the captain who uses his power to humiliate his crew, or the surgeon who vents his irritation by throwing his instruments on the floor or swearing at the theatre sister, are exercising control in a way that asserts ascendancy over, and undermines, the others. From the point of view of the psychological state of the individual who is being controlled, the important variable is not how much control is exercised but whether the control is being used to impose ascendancy and to reduce his personal value. For the purpose of this discussion I propose to define as domination only those acts which are undermining, restricting, or hostile.

Although acceptance and domination may be regarded as separate dimensions, in any actual interaction the two forms of behaviour are, of course, linked. Both domination and rejection reflect hostility, and in any relationship in which there is affective involvement the withdrawal of co-operation or of affection, either by a refusal to fulfil the appropriate role or by the denial of the direct expression of affection, provides one of the major weapons whereby control is exercised. Such withdrawal of affect plays a large part in both parent–child interactions and in the marriage relationship. Sexual behaviour does not differ from other expressive behaviour, in that it may be either co-operative, expressing giving and acceptance, or controlling,

H 113

expressing manipulation, rejection, or punishment. The hostile content of frigidity, for example, is well known clinically. Other means whereby control may be exercised, even in close relationships which include positive affective bonds, are direct domineering, the use of symptoms of illness, the imposition of dependency, or the use of dependency to arouse guilt in the other.

Intensity of interaction provides in theory a third dimension in the analysis of the content of a relationship. It is, however, a dimension which is not fully independent of either acceptance–rejection or domination–submission, for intensity can be related to either domination or affection, and detachment can be seen as a weapon of, or a defence against, control, or as a form of rejection.

(b) Goals and rewards of relationships

Whether a given act is sensed by the other as accepting, rejecting, dominating, or submissive depends not only upon the act itself but also upon the context in which it is committed, in particular upon the relative roles of the two individuals concerned. Psychiatry is primarily concerned with relationships where the response of the other is an important goal of behaviour, that is to say with relationships with affective goals internal to the relationship. Not all relationships are of this sort. For example, the co-operation between a railway engine driver and a signalman is necessary for the train to go through, but beyond the mutual trust involved it is in no sense an affective relationship between the two individuals; the driver could in fact trust an electronic device equally. Two climbers roped together on a difficult rock face are similarly working towards a common goal; though they are likely to be united by a strong bond of trust, this may be relevant only to the particular task of climbing the mountain. Playing a duet, being a doctor, or cleaning a sewer are all rewarded by society with pay and status, and also in varying degrees by the appreciation of the audience, patient, or customer. To be a parent, husband, or wife is also to fulfil a role which is socially determined and socially rewarded, but here the affective rewards of being accepted, loved, and rewarded by the other are of more crucial significance. From the psychiatric point of view an individual is mainly vulnerable to rejection from someone whose acceptance is valued, and can be restricted only by someone whose power is acknowledged. For most people this means that the acceptance and control experienced in their immediate family relationships are central to their psychological stability.

(c) The balance of relationships

Another aspect of the assessment of relationships is that of balance. Co-operative relationships may be reciprocal and equal in that each provides for the other much the same as is provided in return, or they may be unequal but complementary in that one may derive different rewards or satisfactions from those derived by the other but both receive satisfaction. Thus one partner may be nurturant and the other dependent, or one may derive most satisfaction from the internal affective rewards and the other from the external, socially determined rewards. It is also important to recognize that in relationships between adults that appear to lack balance and reciprocity both partners, including, for example, those who are suffering or who appear to be victims, are at some level 'choosing' to be involved.

(d) The roots of interpersonal behaviour

As suggested above, psychiatry is mainly concerned with close personal relationships in which the response of the other provides the main reward. Parents provide the first source of acceptance, and the acceptance they grant is, inevitably, incomplete and conditional. In seeking to meet the conditions for parental acceptance the child becomes 'socialized', but he may, if these conditions are extreme or deviant, also acquire a structure of assumptions, expectations, and fantasies that influence all his subsequent relationships. Whether the lessons learnt in the course of this childhood quest for acceptance are described in terms of learning theory, self theory, personal construct theory, or in terms of internalized objects, it can be agreed that something is carried over into adult life which may be manifest, for example, in the need to placate, submit to, or dominate others, in a need to resemble or differ from one or other parent, in a search for punishment, or in an inability to trust any potential source of love. Moreover, the assumptions learnt in childhood may be so ingrained that evidence that contradicts them may not be perceived; and indeed it seems that the need to provoke their confirmation may become a major behavioural drive.

A relationship between two adults therefore becomes a complex interaction in which each sees himself and the other partly in terms

115

of present reality and present roles, but partly through a filter of assumptions, expectations, and fantasies derived from childhood. To the extent that fantasy and reality needs contradict each other, and to the extent that the role ascribed or fantasied by one for the other conflicts with the role sought by the other, communication becomes difficult and conflict probable.

An adult in a relationship, though to an extent at the mercy of his childhood impressions, can modify his view of himself and others by referring to other past experiences and to present reality. The child, on the other hand, has virtually no possibility of escape from his family, and no other certainty of himself against which to test the virtue or reality of the roles he is expected to play by his parents. This being so, family therapy aimed at saving or helping the child must be based upon the recognition of the parents' unconscious investment in the child and of the roles ascribed to the child in the family group. The normal child reaches maturity through successive role assignments in the family and through successive revisions of the balance of his dependence and autonomy. The child who has become the vehicle for his parents' neurotic needs may have this process halted or distorted, sometimes to an extreme degree. The processes described in the families of schizophrenics by writers such as Lidz and Lidz (1949), Brody (1959), Dysinger (1961), and Laing and Esterson (1964) are of widespread occurrence in less extreme forms, and it seems likely that they are important antecedents of much psychological disturbance apart from their possible relevance to schizophrenia.

The sources of rejecting or dominating behaviour in parents are themselves in turn rooted in childhood, as indicated above. The parent with low self-acceptance may be unable to give to his child or may become dependent upon the child. A parent may demonstrate projection, punishing bad aspects of himself or herself in the child, or a parent may make unrealistic demands upon the child through idealization or over-identification. The parent whose sole satisfaction is derived from the parent role may not allow a child to grow up. Between unhappily married couples displacement of hostility onto the child may occur, the deficiencies of the spouse being punished in the child. Within the whole family group the child may further be used in various ways, for example as the ally of one parent against the other, or as a bridge between the parents, or as the family scapegoat.

Understanding the network of unconscious feeling within a family

116

is a prerequisite of treatment, but it demands closer contact than that provided by research interviewing. Our rating of 'neurotic involvement' provided an indication of Miss Hamilton's recognition of this type of parent–child interaction, as the following case histories indicate, but in most cases longer contact would have been required to unravel the whole tapestry.

Family diagnosis illustrations – the diagnosis of relationships

(i) The Peters family
Family composition: Father, a second-hand-car dealer, aged 45; mother aged 34; Yvonne aged 11; William aged eight; Brian aged seven.
Family ratings: The father's childhood home was intact and emotionally secure (1). Mother had experienced the loss of a parent and emotional disturbance (6). Their C.M.I. scores were: father 32, mother 46. The marital rating was open conflict (4). On the Macfarlane scales, all the children scored in the upper range: Yvonne 23, William 33, Brian 23. Both parents had numerous contacts (4), and all the children had several friends (2). Family unity was rated as major differences (3). Mother's household management was efficient but flexible (2). As regards child-rearing attitudes, mother's consistency varied with moods (3), her acceptance was low, domination high, and neurotic involvement present. The father's consistency was rated totally unpredictable (5). Acceptance was low, domination low, neurotic involvement present. Children's prospects were rated: Yvonne uncertain (3), William and Brian poor (4).
Diagnostic formulation (relationships): This was a disturbed family with both the father and the eldest son in trouble with the law for antisocial behaviour. The marriage was one in which communication was poor and in which there were many serious stresses. There was no evidence of domination of one by the other, but neither the husband nor the wife received adequate emotional support from the other, and this had led to a mutual detachment and a reliance upon satisfactions found outside the home. As regards the children, the father was weak and inconsistent as a source of discipline, uncertain as a source of affection, and inadequate and socially deviant as an identification figure. The mother was inconsistent as a disciplinarian and also as a source of love, although she was basically a warm

117

person. With Yvonne she was reasonably accepting, while with William she alternated between affection and exasperation and with Brian she was often frustrated by his lack of response. The information was insufficient to provide a full understanding of the patients' personalities or of the psychodynamics of these relationships, but there was evidence that mother's relationship with William, in particular, contained elements of both projection and displacement.

(ii) The Mitchell family

Family composition: Father aged 40, an insurance salesman; mother aged 33; Jonathan and David, twins aged seven.

Family ratings: Father's childhood experience was of poverty but he had been emotionally secure (2). Mother's childhood home was intact with major emotional disturbance (5). C.M.I. scores: father 20, mother 24. The marital rating was stresses contained (3). Macfarlane scores: both children scored in the lower range (13). The parents showed some social participation outside the family (3), and the children had several friends (2). Mother's household management was efficient but flexible (2). Family unity was rated 3 (major differences). Child-rearing attitudes: in mother, consistency varied with mood (3), her acceptance was adequate, domination high, and she showed neurotic involvement with the children. Father was consistent but flexible (1), his acceptance was low and his domination was intermediate.

Diagnostic formulation (relationships): The parents' marriage was an uneasy alliance, in which neither provided any significant degree of emotional support for the other. Since the mother's discovery of an infidelity some years before, no real attempt at restoration had been made. Father derived some satisfaction from his work, whereas mother relied upon her own family, and upon her involvement with the children; she had also needed support (general practice psychotherapy) and medication. Both parents provided a reasonably secure source of acceptance and of authority to the children, but the rift between the parents, and the mother's over-involvement with, and dependence upon, the twins were likely to become increasingly damaging.

CONCLUSION

In this chapter an attempt has been made to formulate some of the features of the family that are of relevance in psychiatry. While it is sometimes valid to regard the family as an autonomous unit – as a small social system or as a sub-group of a larger kinship network and in turn of a sub-culture or a society – psychiatric interest inevitably returns to the individual within the family and, in the case of preventive psychiatry, to the individual child. The object of 'family diagnosis' is not, therefore, to make of the family a new organism with its own rules and needs, but rather to place the individuals' symptoms in the context of the network of forces to which they are related. These forces, in turn, can only be adequately understood in terms of individual psychodynamics.

Individual diagnosis in psychiatry is still too often made as if psychiatric disorder was a parallel phenomenon to somatic disorder. For many purposes it may be more valuable to look upon much psychiatric illness as a form of, or as a failure of, communication between the individual and those around him. While family diagnosis has many weaknesses, due both to the complexity of the phenomena and to the unfamiliarity of the field, the inadequacy of a purely individual approach to the phenomena of psychiatric disturbance is becoming increasingly apparent.

The children's social participation rating

1. Active in clubs, etc.
2. Has several contemporary-age-group friends.
3. Plays with family only or single friends.
4. Solitary, but with satisfying pursuits.
5. Solitary with no resources.

The mothers' household management rating

1. Highly organized, rigid routine.
2. Efficient but flexible.
3. Happy-go-lucky, efficient in some areas, haphazard in others.
4. Disorganized.

The family unity rating

1. United family.
2. Minor differences, minor alliances.
3. Major differences, major alliances, or locked in combat.
4. Fragmented family with individuals going their own ways.

The children's prospects rating

1. Good.
2. Satisfactory.
3. Uncertain.
4. Poor.
5. Very poor.

CHAPTER 10

Consultation and Treatment

Without doubt no man who sees only with his eyes can know anything of what has been here described. It is for this reason that I have called them obscure, even as they have been judged to be by the art. Their obscurity, however, does not mean that they are our masters, but as far as is possible they have been mastered, a possibility limited only by the capacity of the sick to be examined and of researchers to conduct research.

Hippocrates, *The art* (translated by W. H. S. Jones)

The C.M.I. scores of the parents and the Macfarlane ratings of the children provide measures of the prevalence of neurotic symptoms in the population. The present chapter deals with the relationship between the scores on these instruments, and the medical response sought by the patients and provided by myself as the family doctor and by the specialist psychiatric services. Clearly, my own pattern of response and my referral habits were not typical. The fact that I set aside four or five hours weekly outside surgery time for psychiatric consultations placed me among the more psychiatrically active general practitioners, despite which fact my referral rate to psychiatric outpatient departments was higher than that of my less psychiatrically orientated partners in the practice, and the overall psychiatric referral rate of my partnership was in turn six times the rate recorded for the county of Buckinghamshire (6 per 1,000 per year), as reported by Kessel and Shepherd (1962). In the case of children, my referral rate to child guidance clinics was relatively high, being ten times the national rate reported by Douglas and Mulligan (1961). Nonetheless, however idiosyncratic my own practice may have been, this investigation can still provide some evidence as to the factors associated with consultation or non-consultation in groups with similar evidence of neurosis according to the C.M.I. or the Macfarlane ratings.

FACTORS ASSOCIATED WITH CONSULTATION
AND REFERRAL IN ADULTS

In the first place it can be recorded that rising C.M.I. scores were associated with higher consultation rates, with a higher rate of selection for long appointments outside surgery hours, and with a higher hospital referral rate. These associations are demonstrated in *Figure 1*, which refers to the period of five years preceding the survey interviews. Any individual who had consulted once, had one long appointment, or had been referred to hospital once during this period counts towards the appropriate total. This graph shows an increase in all these measures with increasing C.M.I. score. It is noticeable that there was a marked sex difference in the percentage with a G.P. consultation or a G.P. long appointment, men showing much lower rates at each C.M.I. level. The percentage of men referred to hospital, however, was only slightly lower than the percentage of women at each level, although the lower mean scores for men meant that the total number of men referred remained lower than that of women.

It is apparent from this graph that among those with C.M.I. scores of 31 + there remained about one in five women and one in three men who had gone for five years without ever presenting with their neurotic symptoms for medical advice. This finding could be interpreted either as meaning that the C.M.I. score is only approximately related to neurotic 'illness' and that the majority of high C.M.I. scorers remain 'well' with no need of doctors; or as meaning that many people are 'ill' without attending the doctor. This raises the question of defining illness. To define illness as a condition for which people seek medical advice can be convenient for some purposes, but it begs the question when one is dealing with a widespread, variable disorder, such as neurosis, to which both medical and public attitudes show major changes.

This argument can perhaps be expounded by analogy. In some ways, 'neuroticism' could be compared with hypertension. For every patient whose high blood pressure has been diagnosed there are others in the community with pressures at similar levels who remain

122

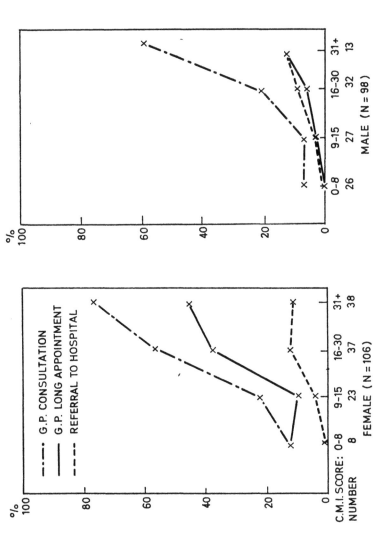

FIGURE 1 RELATION OF C.M.I. SCORES OF PARENTS
TO CONSULTATION AND REFERRAL

undiagnosed. The rate of hypertensive illness recorded in a community will therefore vary, according to the rate at which people seek medical examination and according to the willingness of doctors to use sphygmomanometers, and also according to the levels of pressure regarded as evidence of disease. Public education, or the adoption by doctors of different criteria of normality, or the development of case-finding techniques, could clearly profoundly alter the rate of hypertensive 'illness' in such community without altering, in fact, the number of people with high blood pressures. The same may well be true of neurosis. In other respects, perhaps, neurosis should be compared with leprosy, for it remains a condition which to some extent penalizes the individual or exposes him to shame or ridicule; readiness to consult is reduced by these attitudes and the rate of 'illness' is therefore apparently lowered.

Unfortunately, in the case of those with high C.M.I. scores we do not possess any independent criterion of severity by means of which the consulters and non-consulters can be compared. We can, however, compare them in respect of certain associated factors which might be considered to have a bearing on consultation. Three factors were selected for study: the marital rating, the spouse's neuroticism, and the degree of contact with the extended family. These three factors were selected to test the hypothesis that high-scoring individuals with satisfactory close personal relationships would be less liable to need support from the doctor. The individuals were classified according to the C.M.I. score into three groups (10–15, 16–30, and 31+), and according to whether or not they had consulted during the previous five years; these three groups were further divided as follows: (1) According to the marital rating. (2) According to the spouse's neuroticism (in the case of wives, a score of 31+ on the C.M.I. and in the case of husbands the criterion of 'minimal neurosis' being used). (3) According to the degree of contact with their own parents, those having contact monthly or more often being separated from those with less frequent or no contact. No relationship was found between neurosis in the spouse or contact with own parents and consultation rates, but individuals with poor marital ratings were more likely to consult (*Table 32*). Taking the whole population, irrespective of C.M.I. score, this association is significant for mothers ($\chi^2 = 6.0$, $p < 0.02$) and significant at the

10 per cent level for fathers ($\chi^2 = 2\cdot8$). A similar trend was apparent in respect of hospital referral, but numbers were small and not significant.

TABLE 32 CONSULTATION WITH G.P. FOR NEUROSIS RELATED TO THE MARITAL RATING AND C.M.I. SCORE

		Mothers					*Fathers*		
C.M.I.		*Consulta-tion for*	*Marital rating* *Satis-*				*Consulta-tion for*	*Marital rating* *Satis-*	
score	*Number*	*neurosis*	*factory*	*Poor*	*Number*		*neurosis*	*factory*	*Poor*
0–15	31	Yes 6	2	4	59		Yes 4	3	1
		No 25	19	6			No 49	30	19
16–30	37	Yes 21	11	10	32		Yes 8	1	7
		No 16	11	5			No 24	14	10
31+	38	Yes 27	7	20	13		Yes 8	3	5
		No 11	3	8			No 5	2	3
Total	106	Yes 54	20	34	98		Yes 20	7	13
		No 52	33	19			No 78	46	32

FACTORS ASSOCIATED WITH CONSULTATION
AND TREATMENT IN CHILDREN

The relationship between the Macfarlane scores and the child's consultation and treatment history is similar to that recorded between the C.M.I. scores of the parents and their consultation and treatment history. The percentage consulting, receiving further treatment in the practice, and being referred to child guidance clinics rises with the score on the Macfarlane ratings, as is seen in *Figure 2*. 'Consultation' included any consultation during the child's lifetime for a psychological or psychosomatic disorder. 'Further action' included all responses beyond an ordinary consultation in surgery – that is to say the giving of a special long appointment to the child or parent, intervention with the school, or referral for a psychiatric opinion; child guidance referral was also plotted separately, these figures including cases referred after the survey up until mid 1963. None of these referrals was directly prompted by the findings of the survey, but it remains possible that the information gathered, which did have the effect of increasing my total referral rate, may have influenced my selection for referral. As no significant differences between

125

boys and girls were found, the figures are given for the two sexes combined. As with the C.M.I. scores for adults, it is seen that even at high score levels there remained a substantial number of children for whom no consultations had ever been sought, though it may be noted that in the highest scoring group (25+) the rate of 'further action' equals the rate of 'consultation': that is to say that every child scoring in this range who had consulted had been considered as needing some further action. In some cases (as is clinically familiar) the general level of family disorganization, or the degree of emotional disturbance of one or other parent, was responsible for the non-consultation or non-referral of the child.

To investigate what parental factors were associated with consultation, further multiple regressions on the factors investigated in relation to Macfarlane scores and school teacher classification (see Chapter 8) were carried out, using consultation as the outcome

FIGURE 2   RELATION OF MACFARLANE SCORES OF CHILDREN
TO CONSULTATION AND REFERRAL

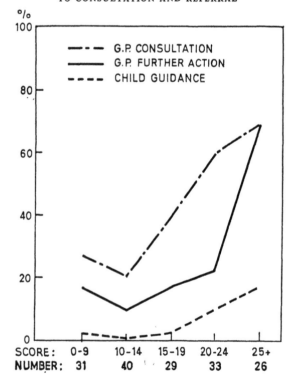

variable. Any consultation during the child's lifetime, for any psychological disorder but not including psychosomatic disorders, was
taken as the criterion. Statistical details of this will be published
elsewhere.

In the case of boys, only two parental factors were significantly
related to consultation, accounting for 18 per cent of the variance,
namely minimal neurosis in mothers, which was negatively associated, and extremes of the fathers' domination (inventory rating)
($p \doteq 0.002$). In the case of girls, consultation was related to mothers'
inconsistency, low domination by interview rating, and to fathers'
inconsistency and high domination by interview rating (percentage
of variance accounted for, 36) ($p < 0.001$). It is of interest that none
of these factors was among those significantly related to the Macfarlane scores or to the teachers' classification, although the total
Macfarlane scores themselves were related to consultation. The range
of factors associated with consultation suggests that uncertainty
about authority may have played a part in leading parents to seek
medical advice, at least in the case of girls. Wolff's (1961) finding of
an association of parents' adverse childhood (parental deprivation)
and parents' psychiatric disturbance with the pre-school children's
referral to child guidance is not repeated in respect of consultation
in this older age-group.

THE SCOPE OF GENERAL PRACTICE PSYCHIATRY

It might be found of interest if the above crude, quantitative account
of the psychiatric treatment of this population were to be supple-
mented with a clinical description and appraisal. The difficulties of
assessing one's own action, in this sphere particularly, are, however
virtually insuperable, and I shall not pretend to measure the effects
of the hundreds of hours represented by the 'further action' and 'long
appointments' of *Figures 1* and *2*. In so far as reading the research
records provided me with an opportunity to look back over what
had been done, my main impression was that major therapeutic
effects were distinctly rare, though support and interpretation through
crises may have prevented deterioration in some cases and perhaps
prevented the establishment of some vicious circles. Most of this
group of parents were, of course, individuals with long-established
personal relationships and at least a working level of adjustment,

and they were therefore not the sort of patient for whom one sets one's therapeutic sights very high. As regards the nature of my psychiatric response, my methods were based initially upon no more than an interest in patients as people and a willingness to see psychological causes for disease. Over the years I gradually reached – through reading, work as a clinical assistant in psychiatry, and, above all, through continued contact with patients – a less naïve, fundamentally eclectic approach, which allowed for drugs and E.C.T. on the one hand and for the analysis of transference on the other, with advice, non-directive counselling, learning-theory techniques, and other methods encompassed in between. Basically, my response was still that of a doctor to the sick individual coming to the surgery, with involvement of the spouse or of the family in treatment occurring in only a minority of cases (although probably more often than is the case with most doctors). The main effect of experience was to make me more cautious in my response to patients' psychiatric demands, less ambitious in my therapeutic aims, and more doubtful and critical of the larger claims made for the power and value of the doctor–patient relationship in general practice. In saying this I am not suggesting that the general neglect of the family doctor's psychiatric role is defensible. Current education, attitudes, and economics combine to create this neglect, but perhaps at times the tendency towards omniscience and omnipotence in the sayings of enthusiasts serves to heighten resistance to psychiatry. My overall opinions on general practice psychotherapy are summarized in the following passage which is taken from a discussion on 'psychotherapy by the non-psychiatrist' (Ryle, 1963):

'Some 30 per cent or so of the population have chronic problems in interpersonal adjustment and will present with chronic or recurrent symptoms of emotional stress and tension. These are the more or less insecure, immature people with only partially-met dependent needs, whose adjustment to life is maintained only at the price of some restriction and of some symptoms. These are people whose adjustment to each other incorporates neurotic mechanisms, often at the cost of some destruction and limitation of personality. It is with this type of patient that general practice psychotherapy is mainly concerned.

The type of help needed by these patients could be described as interpretative support. This may be given in brief interviews in the course of ordinary surgeries, or in special hours outside surgeries, and the ratio of interpretation to support will vary at different times and with different patients. Some patients must be allowed some dependence, some patients will need some advice and some suggestion. With these patients, the general practitioner should attempt to define his role as accepting, non-critical and interested, but he should aim as far as possible to avoid too profound an attachment and dependence on the patients' part. I think it is wrong to believe that these patients inevitably form, or need, an intensive transference relationship with the general practitioner: their neurosis is expressed in their everyday relationships, and treatment can focus upon these relationships. These patients will very seldom fully recover, but the general practitioner can play a part in gradually increasing their self-acceptance and their ability to see themselves and other people more realistically. This sort of psychotherapy may extend over many years, over whole phases of the patient's life, matching in this way the long-term nature of neuroticism. Psychotherapy of this type is a basic and inescapable part of good general practice and is carried out by more general practitioners than would admit to being psychotherapists. However, it is only a partial response and does not take into account the fact that as well as presenting with symptoms, many of these chronic, relatively mild neurotic patients are affecting the lives and emotional health of others, and particularly of their children. It can, I believe, be argued that the treatment of one individual patient may at times imply a type of collusion with a family sickness. The automatic response of the doctor when presented with a patient with symptoms is to attempt to relieve the patient, but the chronic neurotic individual, who is a member of a family group, might often, I believe, be equally helped himself by a therapeutic approach concentrating upon the family group, and such an approach might also offer a chance for preventive psychiatry.'

THE CASE FOR FAMILY-CENTRED TREATMENT

I am not qualified to argue in detail the case for a family-centred approach to psychiatry. Ackerman (1958) in America, and Howells

(1963) in Great Britain, have presented their views and clinical experience, although neither of these authors has gone very far towards establishing on solid evidence the effectiveness of this approach. One of the few English ventures into family-centred casework is described in *The Canford families* (edited by Halmos, 1962). This experiment, unfortunately shortlived, served to demonstrate the value of a non-doctrinaire family-centred approach combined with group work with children in families not accessible to existing types of service. In America Carroll (1962) and Shellow *et al.* (1963) describe clinic experience of treating families with neurotic problems and both find, within limits, such an approach to be effective. Kaffman (1963) sums up his experience of short-term family therapy as follows:

'Therapists played a very active role during both the family and separate interviews, helping to clarify the nature of conscious and pre-conscious family conflicts and utilizing any possible approach leading to a healthier family readjustment. Clinical evidence shows that the effect of alleviation or removal of a disorganising stress situation and pervading anxiety may result in a sound, continued process of improvement even in the absence of prolonged psycho-therapy.'

Bell (1962) has presented a succinct and comprehensive review of family group therapy. He summarizes the therapist's aims as follows:

'. . . to promote social interaction through communication within the family unit, permitting it thereby to experience, appraise, define, and re-order its relational processes. The therapist builds social action on the basis of his own methods of participation. He conducts relationships – now with one, now with two, now with all – in the presence of the others. He disrupts unsatisfactory patterns of relationship as he permits individuals to reaffirm old intentions that have been frustrated. He calls up new intentions. He encourages the family to clarify its goals, to choose more appropriate group goals for the whole family and more suitable personal goals for use in life outside the family's direct involvement. He demonstrates, through the ways individuals relate to him, that within the family there may be:
(a) increased fluidity in communication;
(b) greater flexibility in roles and functions; and
(c) greater discipline in the choice and forms of relationships.

130

He promotes thereby new evaluations within the family of the potentialities and skills of the individual members. He encourages reassessments of the past, of the responsibility for earlier difficulties, of the meaning of symptomatic behaviour, and of the family climate within which it grew. He prevents any family members from evading the implications of their relationships with him and others. He demonstrates forms of relationship that can be transferred to other interactions in the family. This leads the family to the conviction that change is possible and desirable and may bring about a greater measure of behaviour that the family would interpret as positive.'

Family therapy that aims to help the child must assist the parents and the family group to discover a degree of security that can allow the withdrawal of the destructive forces operating upon the child. A family-centred approach can make use of the strengths and resources which are to be found in all but the most disorganized families. The doctor or caseworker can play the part of a catalyst, encouraging good internal reactions, rather than that of an external reagent, as is the case in individual psychotherapy, and will be needed, one may hope, in an appropriately smaller dose. The apparent objectives of family-centred therapy are lower than those of individual psychotherapy, no attempt being made to modify basic personality patterns. If effective, however, it may well be that the preventive impact of such treatment would be greater per man hour of doctor or social worker than more ambitious and intensive forms of treatment.

Had family casework services been available in our population – had Miss Hamilton in fact had a therapeutic brief – we estimated that family casework might have been of value in nearly half of the survey families. For some, family casework would have offered the only possible form of psychiatric intervention: these were usually the most severely disturbed and disrupted families. For others, it would have been seen as a preliminary measure, possibly leading on to child guidance or other forms of treatment. For the majority, however, it would have been a service provided for the family in parallel to my own medical service to individuals in which the caseworker would share the general practitioner's time relationship with the patients – a relationship based upon long-term, non-intensive contact and availability at times of crisis. One way in which the social worker and doctor could work together would be that the doctor's handling of sick individuals would be carried out in the light of the social worker's picture of total family function, the social worker supporting the other members of the family in the face of changed behaviour resulting from the treatment of individuals. We believe that such a service at general practice level might prove both effective and economical, but this can be no more than a belief until this and other therapeutic measures have been subjected to trial.

CHAPTER 11

Evaluation and Conclusions

> It is much more easy to have sympathy with suffering than it
> is to have sympathy with thought.
>
> Oscar Wilde

The study reported in this book was deficient in a large number of
ways, particularly in respect of the validity of the techniques of
recording and rating used. Perhaps some criticism may be forestalled
by acknowledging and apologizing for these deficiencies, which were
most marked in the attempts made to rate intrapersonal behaviour.
We can also, I hope, claim some strengths, of which three are of
particular importance in the context of other work in this field.

The first of these was that we had access to a psychiatrically un-
selected, co-operative population; the literature is heavily sprinkled
with references to the need for data from such populations but it is
strikingly deficient in examples of it. There is little doubt that the
access and co-operation granted to us were the result of the previous
relationship I had established with the families as their general
practitioner. While some clearly found difficulty in adjusting to my
dual role, the majority welcomed the idea of the research and gave
wholehearted co-operation in a way which, I believe, would not have
been achieved by any more impersonal approach. For an inquiry
that investigates the private areas of individual and family life, the
advantages of such an already established relationship outweigh the
inevitable restriction and selection of a population confined to a
single general practice. In view of the importance of surveys of
normal populations in relation to a whole number of problems in
psychiatry, it is to be hoped that this research may serve to underline
the potentiality of general practice as a research field and to bring
nearer the day when general practitioners carrying out academic

133

work in general practice in co-operation with other specialists will cease to be a rarity.

The second strength of our survey was the structure of our team and the good fortune (or skill?) which made our co-operation stimulating and successful. No serious barriers to communication operated between us, perhaps because, although we came from the three separate fields of consultant psychiatry, psychiatric social work, and general practice, we had all had experience overlapping each other's fields.

The third strength was the choice of the whole family as the focus of interest in the survey. We were conducting a survey which was basically exploratory, rather than testing a set of hypotheses, and some might consider the design of the research diffuse in that the associations or theories to be tested were not more rigorously delineated. However, observation and fact-gathering must precede both policy-making and hypothesis-testing. If our research design was weak in some ways, we can claim that such associations as we have demonstrated between different family factors, although they are frequently inconclusive, are presented in the context of a range of other relevant family and individual variables, and are hence less likely to be misleading than studies of falsely isolated and simplified variables.

In this final chapter I propose to discuss the findings of our survey in relation to other work in the field under three headings:

1. Psychological disturbance in adults, children, and families.
2. Medical response to the problem of neurosis.
3. Research needs.

THE RATES OF PSYCHOLOGICAL DISTURBANCE
IN ADULTS, CHILDREN, AND FAMILIES

As far as neurosis in adults is concerned, the findings in the parents of our families are in line with a number of recent epidemiological surveys. A previous study of the practice (Ryle, 1960) showed an annual consultation rate for neurosis of the same order as the rates of 'conspicuous psychiatric morbidity' found in the South London practice study carried out by Kessel (1960) and in line also with the many other general practice studies reviewed by Kessel and Shepherd (1962). The C.M.I. scores in our population are at the average

Evaluation and Conclusions

level of the scores found in a number of other practices by Cooper (see Chapter 2). Scores over 30 are found in many more individuals than consult annually, which suggests that annual consultation rates reflect only a part of the 'neurotic iceberg' although, as shown in Chapter 11, over a five-year period more than three-quarters of those scoring 31 or more on the Cornell Medical Index had consulted.

This last finding suggests that there may be less need to distinguish between 'neuroticism' and neurosis than is argued by Hare and Shaw (1965). These authors compared M.P.I. neuroticism scores and neurosis diagnosed by the general practitioner over a one-year period with a number of other health and social indices and found differences between the two criteria. Only diagnosed neurosis was correlated with poor physical health and dissatisfaction with the district. This association could, however, be explained as a factor relating to consultation-proneness rather than to the presence or absence of neurotic symptoms. This interpretation is strengthened by the evidence that even M.P.I. neuroticism scores are reflections of current health rather than of a personality trait; thus Lucas *et al.* (1965) found the scores accurate current indicators but poor predictors of psychiatric illness in students, and Coppen and Metcalfe (1965) showed significant changes in M.P.I. scores on recovery from depressive illness.

Cooper and Brown (personal communication) found a tendency for the proportion of the population scoring 30 or more on the C.M.I. to rise with age, this rise being due to the A–L ('organic') section of the form and being accompanied by a drop in the more directly psychiatric M–R scores. The evidence for any marked fall in the rate of neurosis with age is small. Kay *et al.* (1964) found that 31 per cent of a sample of a population aged 65 or over had some functional nervous disorder, mostly neurosis, and they found in this population, as in younger groups, a significantly higher rate in women. Studies from many countries confirm the picture of a high and persistent burden of neurosis in the population, the differences in rates between different studies probably reflecting differing criteria rather than real differences in prevalence (for example Downes and Simon, 1954, and Pasamanick *et al.*, 1957, from the U.S.A.; Strömgren *et al.*, 1961, from Denmark; Bremer, 1951, from Norway; and Lin, 1953, from Formosa. See also the review in Lin and Standley, 1962). Our study has served to indicate how the common neuroses of adults are linked

135

with the conflicts of their parents, and with the disturbances of their children.

Published British evidence on the prevalence of childhood psychological disturbance in normal populations is confined to Douglas and Mulligan's valuable indirect study (Douglas and Mulligan, 1961; Mulligan *et al.*, 1963), which has paid increasing attention to psychological problems, and to Brandon's (1960) unpublished study of a section of the Newcastle 1,000 families survey which found that at least one in five of the child population was disturbed at the age of 11. Bremer's (1951) classic study of a small Norwegian town, which offers many parallels to our own research, showed that over a five-year period one-quarter of the children aged 5–14 years gave evidence of a psychological disturbance. Bremer divided these children into the 'mainly asthenic' and 'mainly aggressive' groups, finding a male preponderance in the latter group which was not apparent in our sample, perhaps due to his higher upper age limit. In America, Lapouse and Monk (1958) investigated a random sample of children aged 6–12 in Buffalo by means of a 200-item structured interview, and found frequencies of a number of specific behaviours which gives an impression of a rate of disturbance similar to that found in our sample.

As regards family disturbance, criteria of broken homes are poorly standardized in the literature, and comparisons are not easy. Using the criterion of loss or absence of one parent (other than in the services) before the age of 15, 20 per cent of the parents of our families came from broken homes and we estimate (Chapter 5) that a similar proportion of the children in our sample will experience broken homes before they reach the age of 15. When we consider that our sample excludes cases of total family breakdown, contains only four Social Class V families, and that the nine non-co-operating families contained a higher proportion of disrupted homes than the sample, our figures are not strikingly lower than those found by Wardle (1960) in his child guidance population. In his sample, 31 per cent (perhaps more) of his parents came from broken homes and 35 per cent of the children did so. While not disagreeing with Wardle's conclusion that children from disrupted families are a particularly vulnerable group, I feel it would be a mistake to exaggerate the role of family disruption in provoking disturbance at the cost of neglecting the many problems of intact families. In our own sample, despite

136

the manifest difficulties of the single-parent family, the children in these families did not score higher on the Macfarlane scales than did the children in intact families.

As regards the relation between illness in different members of the family and other aspects of family life, the main burden of this book has been to demonstrate these associations and no detailed recapitulation is called for here. At varying levels of validity and sophistication we have demonstrated some relationship between the parents' childhood experiences and adult neuroticism (Chapter 4), between these factors and their marriage relationship (Chapter 5), and between these factors, their child-rearing behaviour, and the emotional health of the children (Chapters 6, 7, 8). It is hoped that these chapters will have served to support the arguments put forward in favour of family-centred diagnosis (Chapter 9).

Epidemiological studies in the field of family psychiatry have been relatively few and far between, but mention should be made of the paper by Buck and Laughton (1959) which demonstrated a relationship between maternal and child neurosis, and of the recent paper by Hare and Shaw (1965) showing this association for fathers. Clinical studies of family sickness are, of course, legion. Perhaps their main lesson for epidemiologists is that the time is overdue for the replacement in research surveys of crude indices of health, personality, and interaction (such as we have used) by measures more subtle and relevant to the complexities of interpersonal behaviour.

MEDICAL RESPONSE TO THE PROBLEM OF NEUROSIS

The responses to neurosis supplied by general practice, by psychiatry, and by social work are all undergoing rapid transition. In general practice, while a considerable proportion of doctors respond to neurosis with pharmacological means (and often with irritated letters to the medical press), there is an increasing willingness to acknowledge the possibilities offered for psychotherapeutic intervention. In psychiatry there is an extension of psychiatric interest and time out of the mental hospitals into the community. In social work, the meeting of the physical needs of the socially and physically handicapped is being increasingly linked with attempts to understand and meet their emotional needs also.

In all these fields it is common experience to find the provision of

137

new services rapidly matched by the discovery of new needs, and it is certain that only the tip of the 'neurotic iceberg' has been exposed. In this sorcerer's apprentice situation, the deployment of resources and the planning of future services is a matter of some urgency, and in this section I intend to put forward my personal views on this subject; views which have been influenced by the findings of our survey but which should clearly be tested against more specifically designed operational research.

It will be clear from the mode of inquiry and presentation of this study that, while we studied psychological disturbance in our population from a clinical viewpoint, we sought constantly to set it in the context of individual's relationships and history, and I think it may be claimed that we have provided some justification for the view of neurosis which regards the individual's world of interpersonal experience as of major importance, and which regards in particular his childhood family as the key group in determining his chances of stability and maturity.

Beyond this, I intend to argue from the assumption that psycho-therapeutic treatment can offer a possibility of correcting the damage done by an adverse childhood, and from the certainty that the provision of individual psychotherapy can never be extended to more than a minority of the neurotic individuals in the community. This being so, there would seem to be a strong case for concentrating the main resources of psychiatry upon young individuals who have not yet become entangled in neurotic adult relationships, for in them personality structure is more fluid and external pressures to remain neurotic are minimal. A prevention-orientated psychiatric service might be well advised to concentrate psychotherapeutic resources upon late childhood, adolescence, and early adult life, leaving the young child in the family and the married adult to an alternative service. This alternative service should, I believe, be a family case-work service preferably based upon general practice under close psychiatric supervision. Its aims would be limited in terms of the individual personality but large in terms of society, namely to help parents to contain their neurosis in ways that are minimally restricting and damaging to the others in the family, and above all in ways that do least harm to the children.

In parallel with this development, I believe that a major re-evaluation of the functions of schools is due. The small, intense, and more or less isolated nuclear family of today gives children a very small range of adults with whom to relate, and in consequence little chance of correcting the false impressions and of escaping the distorting roles imposed by neurotic parents. The schoolteacher could become one stable, reliable figure to such children, but the schoolteacher of today has neither the training and supervision nor the time to fulfil this role, and is often drawn into a role which helps to confirm the child in his neurosis by being driven to intolerance of the acting-out child and grateful acquiescence towards the neurotically inhibited one. The nursery school, especially where family disruption on stress occurs, can clearly play a particularly valuable role and a much wider provision of such schools would seem desirable.

Family casework in general practice, and the encouragement of a more consciously stabilizing or therapeutic role for teachers, are two examples of the dissemination of psychiatric skills among non-psychiatrists. This same process should also occur within other branches of medicine and other professions, particularly in all those branches of the welfare services such as health visiting that have frequent 'grass-roots' contact with families with children. Such a dissemination of psychiatric skills among non-psychiatrists alters, but in no way diminishes, the psychiatrist's importance. While retaining ultimate clinical and research responsibility, the psychiatrist would, however, spend increasing time at the task of helping others step outside the restrictions upon understanding others which are imposed by their own personalities and by their *déformations professionnelles*. The skill of the psychiatrist is to be able to understand and enter into the patient's world in a positive and human way, and it is only by passing this skill on to others that the widespread problems of neurosis can be adequately countered.

Before the psychiatrist can accept this role, he himself may have to lose some of his own preoccupations and step out of his own *déformation professionnelle*, for the roots of psychiatry in medicine make situations other than the structured doctor–patient pair relationship unfamiliar and at times threatening, and suspicion of any dilution of skills is common to all craftsmen. Perhaps the psychiatrist's increasing recognition of the contributions of other behavioural sciences such as psychology and sociology could be extended to inviting their examination of his own profession.

As regards the family doctor, there is hope that an increasing proportion of the younger generation may be able to accept psychiatry as a scientific and respectable branch of medicine, even if the economic conditions of general practice still frustrate any major deployment of time in this field. It is uncertain whether the refusal to recognize neurosis cuts down a family doctor's case-load, but I think the reverse argument that the general-practitioner/psychotherapist radically reduces his case-load by dealing appropriately with his neurotic patients is based more upon optimism than upon evidence. My personal experience of psychiatrically orientated general practice and the findings of our family survey make it clear that the individual general practitioner faces the same problem as society in that increased provision of services leads to increased demand. The correct role of the G.P. of the future, in my view, will be to use his unique and trusted access to the family to be a real family doctor in the field of psychiatry. He must be far more prepared to move away from his individual doctor–patient relationship, however gratifying it may be, and more prepared to intervene in the system of family relationships which underly the sickness of the different individuals. This is not to say that his main role may not continue to be the support of individuals, but this support should be carried out with more skill and sophistication as psychiatric supervision is increasingly utilized and never at the cost of ignoring the family implications of individual sickness. To achieve this would probably involve psychiatric supervision at seminar level and co-operation and teamwork with family caseworkers on a day-to-day basis.

In concluding this section, I would re-emphasize that, however impractical or open to improvement my particular suggestions may seem, the deficiencies and inappropriateness of our present services are not open to question. We are witnessing a growing acknowledgement of the role of psychiatry which threatens to widen still further the gap between evident needs and promise, on the one hand, and achievement and provision of services, on the other. The evaluation of different forms of professional response and some serious research into the social trends relative to psychiatry, general practice, and social work is surely overdue.

Apart from investigations into the role of genetics and of physical injury and disease, the study of the aetiology of psychiatric disturbance must consist mainly of investigating associations between factors in the environment and psychological disturbance in individuals. Clinical studies and case histories can suggest associations but, experimentation being impracticable, only epidemiological methods can test hypotheses. However, the environmental factors studied must be relevant ones, and social psychiatry, up to the present time, has concerned itself very little with the intimate emotional factors which clinical experience indicates as having the greatest significance for the individual's psychological health. The situation is well summarized by Kreitman (1964):

'Over the last few decades social psychiatry has demonstrated correlations between mental illness and certain broad social categories. At the same time clinical, genetic and psychological studies have continued their traditional interest in the illness of the individual. The divergence of these two approaches has left relatively unmapped a large area which is of considerable psychiatric interest; despite much descriptive work, very little has been clearly established (outside genetics) concerning mental illness in the small, closely integrated group, of which the prime example in our culture is the family.'

Post and Wardle (1962) in a review of the neglected field of family neurosis and psychosis, make out a strong case for more research, and comment on work already done as follows: '. . . even those investigations concerned with events and interactions occurring shortly before patients fell ill . . . are unsatisfactory, mainly because they have been prematurely concerned to prove some basic theoretical construct.' Family studies are, of course, likely to be expensive, needing the co-operation of many disciplines and including among them longitudinal investigations, for the effects of a childhood factor or situation may be manifest only many years later. In this area, where important variables are complex and interrelated, experimental design presents a great problem, but at the present time the difficulty of handling data has been much reduced by the availability

141

of computers, and the outstanding problem is the collection of data in a reliable, valid, quantifiable form.

Looking back at the methods used in our own survey, certain obvious improvements suggest themselves. One major fault was that one observer collected the greater part of the data from the parents, so that both respondent and interviewer bias could have accounted for associations found between background and child variables. This could have been overcome by the expensive expedient of having a second interviewer, and this might well have been justifiable. An alternative solution could have been to have placed greater reliance on 'objective' assessments of personality, health, and interaction. While the C.M.I. emerges as a crude but reliable index of neuroticism, neither of the parent-attitude instruments seems to be very satisfactory. Subsequent use of the J.M.P.I. (Furneaux and Gibson, 1961) on some of the children produced exceptionally low N and high L scores, suggesting that in this context defensiveness was too great for reliable results to be expected. It might have been of value to test the children's perception of their parents, rather than relying upon judgement derived from the parents, and a follow-up study of the older children using the Bene-Anthony Family Relations Test (1957) is being carried out. An additional follow-up activity has been the development of a marital patterns test which provides a measure of the level of affection and of the balance of domination–submission. While research activity in the field of family psychiatry is likely to proliferate instruments designed to measure personality and interpersonal behaviour, the clinical interview will undoubtedly remain of central importance. Improving techniques in interviewing and recording, and in estimating observer reliability, can overcome many of the snags of this method.

In the field of aetiological research, therefore, two main tasks are apparent. First, to correct the British neglect of the family in psychiatric research, a task to which our survey has, we hope, made a small contribution; and, second, to develop more reliable tools and means of measurement.

Alongside basic aetiological research there is, as indicated above, an urgent need for investigation into the operation of existing social and medical services. The potential size of the neurotic case-load is such that intelligent planning must concern itself with the public and medical attitudes to, and with the effects of, different kinds of social and professional response, if chaos is not to ensue. We do not know what determines whether a neurotic child or adult consults with the family doctor. We do not know what determines the family doctor's treatment or his referral for psychiatric treatment. We do not know which type of patient benefits from which type of treatment, although we do know that overall results are disappointing even with children with whom hopes of preventive intervention and of cure should be highest (Levitt, 1957). We do not know how treated and untreated patients differ in respect of symptoms or in respect of their effect upon others around them. We do not know what social institutions and what public customs and attitudes provide effective supports for the vulnerable individual. In fact we know all too little about this branch of medical practice and what little we do know offers scant basis for complacency.

Faced with this challenge, are we not still too often content to propose conventional or fashionable solutions; too much like the Canute of the story book, bidding the waves go back, and too little like the probable Canute of history, studying the causes of flooding and encouraging society to build up a system of defences?

References

ACKERMAN, N. W. (1958). *The psychodynamics of family life*. New York: Basic Books.

AINSWORTH, M. D. (1962). In: *Deprivation of maternal care, a reassessment of its effects*. Geneva: World Health Organization, Public Health Papers No. 14.

ANDRY, R. G. (1960). *Delinquency and parental pathology*. London: Methuen.

AUSUBEL, D. P., BALTHAZAR, E. E., ROZENTHAL, I. BLACKMAN, L. S., SCHPOONT, S. H., and WELKOWITZ, J. (1954). Perceived parent attitudes as determinants of children's ego structure. *Child Develop.* 25, 3.

BALDWIN, A. L. (1948). Socialization and the parent-child relationship. *Child Develop.* 19 (3) 127.

BARNES, J. A. (1963). Some ethical problems in modern field work. *Brit. J. Sociol.* 14 (2) 118.

BECKER, W. L. (1960). The relationship of factors in parental rating of self and each other to the behaviour of kindergarten children as rated by mothers, fathers and teachers. *J. consult. Psychol.* 24 (6) 507.

BELL, J. E. (1962). Recent advances in family group therapy. *J. Child Psychol. Psychiat.* 3, 1.

BENE, E. and ANTHONY, J. (1957). *Manual for the family relation test*. London: National Foundation for Educational Research.

BERNARD, C. (1957). *An introduction to the study of experimental medicine*. Translated by H. C. Green. New York: Dover; London: Constable.

BOWLBY, J. (1952). *Maternal care and mental health*. Geneva: World Health Organization, Monograph Series No. 2.

BRANDON, S. (1960). An epidemiological study of maladjustment in childhood. D.M. thesis. Durham University.

BREMER, J. (1951). Social psychiatric investigation of a small community in Northern Norway. *Acta Psychiat. Scand., Suppl.* 62.

BRODMAN, K., ERDMANN, A. J., LORGE, I., and WOLFF, H. G. (1949). The C.M.I. – an adjunct to medical interview. *J. Amer. med. Ass.* 140 (6) 530.

BRODMAN, K., ERDMANN, A. J., LORGE, I., and WOLFF, H. G. (1951). The C.M.I. health questionnaire as a diagnostic instrument. *J. Amer. med. Ass.* 145 (3) 152.

BRODMAN, K., ERDMANN, A. J., LORGE, I., GERSHENSEN, C. P., and WOLFF, H. G. (1952). The C.M.I. health index; the evaluation of emotional disturbance. *J. clin. Psychol.* 8, 119.

BRODMAN, K., ERDMANN, A. J., LORGE, I., WOLFF, H. G., and DEUTSCHER-BERGER, J. (1954). The C.M.I. health questionnaire; the prediction of

144

psychosomatic and psychiatric disabilities in army training. *Amer. J. Psychiat.* **111** (1) 37.

BRODY, W. N. (1959). Some family operations and schizophrenia. *Arch. gen. Psychiat. (Chic.)* **1**, 379.

BROWN, A. C., and FRY, J. (1962). The C.M.I. health questionnaire in the identification of neurotic patients in general practice. *J. psychosom. Res.* **6**, 185.

BUCK, C., and LAUGHTON, K. (1959). Family patterns of illness. *Acta Psychiat. Scand.* **34**, 165.

CARROLL, E. J. (1960). Treatment of the family as a unit. *Pennsylv. med. J.* **63** (57) 62.

CARSTAIRS, G. M. (1958). Some problems of psychiatry in patients from alien cultures. *Lancet* (1) 1217.

CHESS, S., THOMAS, A., BIRCH, H. G., and HERTZIG, M. (1960). Implications of a longitudinal study of child development for child psychiatry. *Amer. J. Psychiat.* **117** (5) 434.

CLARKE, A. D. B. and CLARKE, A. M. (1960). Some recent advances in the study of early deprivation. *J. Child Psychol. Psychiat.* **1** (1) 26.

COPPEN, A., and METCALF, M. (1965). Effect of a depressive illness on M.P.I. scores. *Brit. J. Psychiat.* **111**, 236.

CRANDALL, J. and PRESTON, A. (1955). Pattern and levels of maternal behaviour. *Child Develop.* **26** (4) 267.

CULPAN, R. H., DAVIS, B. M., and OPPENHEIM, A. N. (1960). Incidence of psychiatric illness among hospital outpatients. *Brit. Med. J.* **1**, 855.

CUMMING, J. H. (1961). The family and mental disorder, in *Causes of mental disorder – a review of epidemiological knowledge*, 1959. Milbank Memorial Fund.

DAHLSTROM, W. G. (1957). Research in clinical psychology: Factor analytic contributions. *J. clin. Psychol.* **13**, 211.

DICKS, H. V. (1959). Clinical studies in marriage and the family – a symposium on methods. *Proc. Roy. Soc. Med.* **52**, 867.

DOUGLAS, J. W. B., and MULLIGAN, D. G. (1961). Emotional adjustment and educational achievement – the preliminary results of a longitudinal study of a national sample of children. *Proc. Roy. Soc. Med.* **54**, 885.

DOWNES, J., and SIMON, K. (1954). Characteristics of psychoneurotic patients and their families as revealed in a general morbidity study. *Milbank Memorial Fund Quart.* **32**, 42.

DYSINGER, R. H. (1961). The family as the unit of study and treatment. *Amer. J. Orthopsychiat.* **31**, 61.

EPSTEIN, N. B. (1958). Concepts of normality or evaluation of mental health. *Behav. Sci.* **3** (4) 335.

ERIKSON, E. H. (1950). *Childhood and society.* New York: W. W. Norton.

FARIS, R. E. L. and DUNHAM, H. W. (1939). *Mental disorders in urban areas.* Chicago: Univ. of Chicago Press.

FROMM, E. (1963). *Fear of freedom.* London: Routledge and Kegan Paul.

FURNEAUX, W. D. and GIBSON, H. B. (1961). A children's personality inventory designed to measure neuroticism and extraversion. *Brit. J. educ. Psychol.* **31**, 204.

GILDEA, M. C. L., GLIDEWELL, J. C., and KANTOR, M. B. (1961). Maternal

K   145

References

attitudes and general adjustment in school children, in *Parental attitudes and child behavior*. Ed. J. C. Glidewell, Springfield, Ill.: Thomas.

GLIDEWELL, J. C., MENSH, I. N., and GILDEA, M. C. L. (1957). Behavior symptoms in children and degree of sickness. *Amer. J. Psychiat.* **114**, 47.

HALMOS, P. (1962). *The Canford families: a study in social casework and group work*. Sociological Review Monograph No. 6. Keele Univ.

HARE, E. H. (1956). Mental illness and social conditions in Bristol. *J. ment. Sci.* **102**, 349.

HARE, E. H., and SHAW, G. K. (1965). A study in family health: 2. A comparison of the health of fathers, mothers and children. *Brit. J. Psychiat.* **111**, 467.

HAMILTON, M., POND, D. A., and RYLE, A. (1962). Relstion of C.M.I. responses to some social and psychologicol factors. *J. psychosom. Res.* **6**, 157.

HENRY, J. (1951). Family structure and the transmission of neurotic behavior. *Amer. J. Orthopsychiat.* **21**, 800.

HEWITT, L. E., and JENKINS, R. L. (1946). *The fundamental patterns of maladjustment*. Springfield, Ill.: Michigan Child Guidance Institute.

HOGGART, R. (1958). *The uses of literacy*. Harmondsworth: Penguin Books.

HOLLINGSHEAD, A. B., and REDLICH, F. C. (1958). *Social class and mental disorder*. New York: Wiley.

HOWELLS, J. G. (1963). *Family psychiatry*. London and Edinburgh: Oliver & Boyd.

INGHAM, H. V. (1949). A statistical study of family relationships in psychoneurosis. *Amer. J. Psychiat.* **106** (2) 91.

KAFFMAN, M. (1963). Short-term family therapy. *Family process* **2** (2) 216.

KAGAN, J. (1956). The child's perception of the parent. *J. abnorm. soc. Psychol.* **52**, 257.

KAY, D. W. K., BEAMISH, P., and ROTH, M. (1964). Old age mental disorders in Newcastle-upon-Tyne. *Brit. J. Psychiat.* **110**, 146.

KESSEL, W. I. N., and SHEPHERD, M. (1962). Neurosis in hospital and general practice. *J. ment. Sci.* **108** (453) 159.

KESSEL, W. I. N. (1960). Psychiatric morbidity in a London general practice. *Brit. J. prev. soc. Med.* **14**, 16.

KREITMAN, N. (1964). The patient's spouse. *Brit. J. Psychiat.* **110**, 159.

LAING, R. D. and ESTERSON, A. (1964). *Sanity, madness, and the family*. London: Tavistock Publications; New York: Basic Books.

LAPOUSE, R. and MONK, M. A. (1959). Fears and worries in a representative sample of children. *Amer. J. Orthopsychiat.* **29**, 803.

LEVITT, E. E. (1957). Results of psychotherapy with children – an evaluation. *J. consult. Psychol.* **21** (3) 189.

LEWIS, H. (1954). *Deprived children*. London: O.U.P.

LIDZ, R. W., and LIDZ, T. (1949). The family environment of schizophrenic patients. *Amer. J. Psychiat.* **106**, 332.

LIN, T. (1953). A study of the incidence of mental disorder in Chinese and other cultures. *Psychiatry* **16**, 313.

LIN, T., and STANDLEY, C. C. (1962). *The scope of epidemiology in psychiatry*. World Health Organization, Public Health Papers No. 16.

146

References

LUCAS, C. J., KELVIN, R. P., and OJHA, A. B. (1965). The psychological health of the pre-clinical medical student. *Brit. J. Psychiat.* **111**, 473.

MACFARLANE, J. W., ALLEN, L., and HONZIK, M. P. (1954). *A developmental study of the behavior problems of normal children between twenty-one months and fourteen years.* University of California publications in child development, Vol. 2. Berkeley and Los Angeles: Univ. of Calif. Press.

MICHAEL, C. M., MORRIS, D. P., and SOZOKON, E. (1957). Follow-up studies of shy withdrawn children. II. Relative incidences of schizophrenia. *Amer. J. Orthopsychiat.* **27**, 331.

MORRIS, H. H., ESCOLL, P. J., and WEXLER, R. (1956). Aggressive behavior disorders in childhood. *Amer. J. Psychiat.* **112**, 991.

MOWRER, O. H. (1950). *Learning theory and personality dynamics.* New York: Ronald.

MOWRER, O. H. (1953). *Psychotherapy theory and research.* New York: Ronald.

MULLIGAN, D. G., DOUGLAS, J. W. B., HAMMOND, W. A., and TIZARD, J. (1963). Delinquency and symptoms of maladjustment. The findings of a longitudinal study. *Proc. Roy. Soc. Med.* **56**, 1083.

NORRIS, V. (1959). Mental illness in London. London: Maudsley Monograph No. 6.

ØDEGAARD, Ø. (1945). Distribution of mental diseases in Norway. *Acta psychiat. neurolog.* **20**, 247.

ØDEGAARD, Ø. (1956). The incidence of psychoses in various occupations. *Int. J. soc. Psychiat.* **2**, 85.

O'NEAL, P., and ROBINS, L. N. (1958). Childhood patterns predictive of adult schizophrenia. *Amer. J. Psychiat.* **115** (5) 385.

PARSONS, T. and BALES, R. F. (1955). *Family socialization and interaction process.* Glencoe, Illinois: Free Press.

PASAMANICK, B., ROBERTS, D. W., LEMKAU, P. V., and KROEGER, D. E. (1957). Survey of mental disease in an urban population. *Amer. J. publ. hlth,* **47** (8) 923.

PETURSSON, E. (1961). A study of parental deprivation and illness in 291 psychiatric patients. *Int. J. soc. Psychiat.* **7** (2) 97.

PHILP, A. F. (1963). *Family failure: a study of 129 families with multiple problems.* London: Faber and Faber.

PITFIELD, M., and OPPENHEIM, A. N. (1964). Child rearing attitudes of mothers of psychotic children. *J. Child Psychol. Psychiat.* **5**, 51.

POND, D. A., HAMILTON, M., and RYLE, A. (1963). Marriage and neurosis in a working class population. *Brit. J. Psychiat.* **109**, 592.

POST, F., and WARDLE, J. (1962). Family neurosis and family psychosis. *J. ment. Sci.* **108**, 147.

PRINGLE, M. L. I. C., and BOSSIO, V. (1960). Early prolonged separation and emotional maladjustment. *J. Child Psychol. Psychiat.* **1**, 37.

ROE, A., and SIEGELMAN, M. (1963). A parent-child relations questionnaire *Child Develop.* **34**, 355.

ROGERS, C. R. (1951). *Client-centred therapy.* Boston: Houghton Mifflin.

ROSENTHAL, M. J. (1962). The syndrome of the inconsistent mother. *Amer. J. Orthopsychiat.* **32**, 637.

References

RUTTER, H., BIRCH, H. G., THOMAS, A., and CHESS, S. (1964). Temperamental characteristics in infancy and the later development of behaviour disorders. *Brit. J. Psychiat.* **110**, 651.

RYLE, A. (1960). The neuroses in a general practice population. *J. Coll. gen. Pract.* **3**, 313.

RYLE, A., and HAMILTON, M. (1962). Neurosis in 50 married couples. *J. ment. Sci.* **108**, 454.

RYLE, A. (1963). Psychotherapy by the non-psychiatrist. *Proc. Roy. Soc. Med.* **56**, 834.

RYLE, A., POND, D. A., and HAMILTON, M. (1965). The prevalence and patterns of emotional disturbance in children of primary age. *J. Child Psychol. Psychiat.* **6**, 101.

SCHAEFER, E. S. (1961). Converging conceptual models for maternal behavior and for child behavior, in *Parental attitudes and child behavior*. edit. J. C. Glidewell. Springfield, Ill.: Thomas.

SEWELL, W. H. (1952). Infant training and the personality of the child. *Amer. J. Sociol.* **58**, 150.

SHELLOW, R. S., BROWN, B. S., and OSBERG, J. W. (1963). Family group therapy in retrospect: four years and sixty families. *Family Process* **2** (1) 52.

SPIEGEL, J. P., and BELL, N. W. (1959). The family of the psychiatric patient. In: *American Handbook of Psychiatry*, edit. S. Arieti. New York: Basic Books.

SPIEGEL, J. P. (1957). The resolution of role conflict within the family. *Psychiatry* **20**, 1.

STRÖMGREN, E., SØRENSEN, A., JOEL-NIELSEN, N., BILLE, M., FLYGENRING, J., and HELGASON, T. (1961). Frequency of depressive states within geographically delimited population groups. *Acta Psychiat. Scand., Suppl.* 162.

THARP, R. G. (1963). Psychological patterning in marriage. *Psychol. Bull.* **60**, 2.

WARDLE, C. J. (1961). Two generations of broken homes in the genesis of conduct and behaviour disorders in childhood. *Brit. med. J.* **2**, 349.

WHITEHORN, J. C. (1962). A working concept of maturity of personality. *Amer. J. Psychiat.* **119** (3) 197.

WILSON, H. (1962). *Delinquency and child neglect.* London: Allen & Unwin.

WINCH, R. F. (1958). *Mate selection.* New York: Harper.

WOLFF, S. (1961). Social and family background of pre-school children with behaviour disorders attending a child guidance clinic. *J. Child Psychol. Psychiat.* **2**, 260.

WOOTTON, B. (1962). In: *Deprivation of maternal care, a reassessment of its effects.* World Health Organization, Public Health Papers No. 14.

YOUNG, M., and WILLMOTT, P. (1962) *Family and kinship in East London.* Harmondsworth: Penguin Books.

Subject Index

Author Index

Author Index

Milton Keynes UK
Ingram Content Group UK Ltd.
UKHW022049141024
449569UK00031B/1565